NURSING THEORY

NURSING THEORY

A Practical Tool for the Advanced Practice Nurse in the Post Pandemic Era

Kerrie Coleman

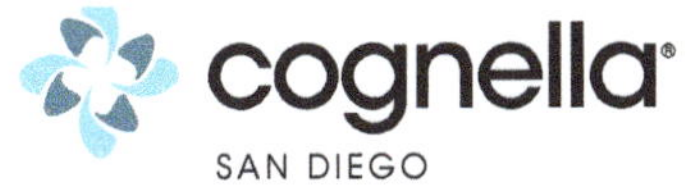

Bassim Hamadeh, CEO and Publisher
Amanda Martin, Executive Publisher
Amy Smith, Associate Editorial Manager
Jeanine Rees, Production Editor
Jess Estrella, Senior Graphic Designer
Kara Tatum, Licensing Coordinator
Natalie Piccotti, Director of Marketing
Kassie Graves, Senior Vice President, Editorial

Printed in the United States of America.

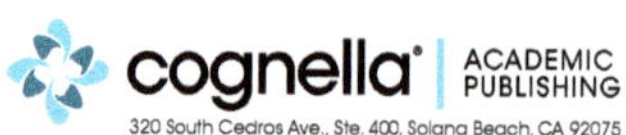

Brief Contents

Detailed Contents

Preface

Nursing Theory: A Practical Tool for Advanced Practice Nurses in the Post-Pandemic Era is an essential book to any master's or doctoral nursing student. The book offers practical, real-world applications of nursing theory to address major health care challenges since the COVID-19 pandemic. As health care delivery has made drastic transitions during and since the pandemic, advanced practice nurses are in an exceptional position to adapt, adopt, and align practice to the core values of who we are as nursing professionals. As nursing theory has been a foundation to defining, prescribing, and predicting the nursing profession, it is time theory is perceived as fluid and dynamic in nature to enhance and synergize nursing practice. This book offers a unique perspective by integrating an extended definition of an advanced practice nurse as clinicians, leaders, and educators. From this three-pronged view, nursing theory becomes a daily tool to meet the growing needs of patients, staff, and students.

The book offers guided application of metacognition as an essential skill in nursing, and through metacognition the student will explore nursing theory from the lens of the nursing metaparadigm: health, environment, person, and nurse. As each section of the book will offer concept definitions and learning objectives, students and professors alike will be engaged in the process of exploring nursing theory in a utilitarian approach. Utilizing critical thinking through reflection will guide students to recognize current nursing trends and align related concepts to theoretical applications, bringing forth a reinvigorated meaning to "theory-guided practice."

A simple, yet practical algorithm is presented with detailed steps for the advanced practice nurse to apply in their individual settings. The algorithm is a culmination of the book's information to guide the student toward using theory in a meaningful and synergistic manner, not only addressing the issue at hand but also in support of the advanced practice nurse's role and contributions as an innovative thinker in this post-pandemic era. As nurses embrace the practice of metacognition, nursing theory becomes less abstract and more of a tool to use anytime, all the time!

Reviewers

Modupe Adewuyi, PhD, MSN/MPH, RN, PHNA-BC, CHES
Kennesaw State University

Dana Clawson, DNS, WHNP, APRN, CNE
Professor of Doctoral Studies
Northwestern State University

Rosemarie Di Mauro Satyshur, PhD, RN
Assistant Professor, Department of Family and Community Health
University of Maryland School of Nursing

Lori Lupe, DNP, CCRN-K(r), NEA-BC
Assistant Professor, Marshall University

Donna Molyneaux, PhD, RN CNE
Professor and Assistant Dean, Graduate Students
Gwynedd Mercy University

PART I

Evolution of a Profession

Nursing is a noble and trusted profession. Even through its evolution from vocational training to a profession with varying levels of preparation and education, the public views nursing as a lifeline and advocate to guide their journey toward health and wellness. Nursing has not only advanced as an art and a science but has adapted to the dynamic nature of health care. Through nursing's journey, nurses have gained a sense of leadership and empowerment to continue its practice of beneficent care and rigorous research to expand nursing knowledge.

As the text opens with a guide to the evolution of nursing, theory will be discussed as the building blocks of nursing's progression. This evolution is guided by theoretical assumptions that highlight phenomena known to the nurse. As the nursing profession adapts to the needs of the person, the nurse, the environment, and health, nurses adopt a systematic approach to form questions framed through the nursing lens. The value of nursing theory cannot be understated as each theory supports nursing thinking and practice.

While the nursing profession continues to grow and modify practice to meet the needs of changing patient demographics, so does the need to revitalize and synthesize nursing theory. As a result of the dynamic health care environment, advanced practice nurse (APN) roles are expanding services to meet the demands of tomorrow's health care challenges. While the APN gains enhanced competencies and knowledge, the APN is equipped to describe and utilize theory through clinical practice, leadership, and education. Theory is the catalyst for generating new knowledge and propelling innovative care practice.

CHAPTER 1

Honoring Its Foundation and Reviving Its Application

Key Terms

Biopsychosocial: Term referring to the holistic approach to nursing focused on one's physical, psychological, and spiritual needs.

Health equity: The state in which everyone has a fair and just opportunity to attain their highest level of health.

Hermeneutic: A method of theory interpretation.

Holistic nursing care: Holistic describes "whole person care," often acknowledging body-mind-spirit.

Interpersonal relations (theory): The interpersonal relations theory posits the assumption that what goes on between people can be noticed, studied, explained, understood, and, if detrimental, changed.

Nursing metaparadigm: A "gestalt or total world view ... that serves as a way of organizing perceptions" (Bender, 2018, p. 1).

Nursing theory guided practice (NTGP): To guide practice by helping nurses clarify their values and beliefs about human health processes and seeking an awareness of patient care approaches.

Paradigm: Specific to nursing as a nursing model or a shared (nursing) view.

Psychodynamic nursing: The goal of psychodynamic nursing is to help understand one's own behavior, help others identify felt difficulties, and apply principles of human relations to the problems that come up at all experience levels.

Social determinants of health (SDOH): Conditions in the places where people live, learn, work, and play that affect a wide range of health risks and outcomes.

Introduction

Nursing theory has been a staple in nursing curricula for decades, and yet it can be a subject matter that heightens students and nurses' anxiety level. Considering this apprehension, nursing theory is proposed as a living tool for the nurse to use to guide practice; hence the concept of nursing theory guided practice (NTGP). Theory holds certain assumptions. Theory is foundational; it describes, it predicts, and it explains (Chinn & Jacobs, 1978). Each assumption contributes to understanding what nursing is and what it does. During the post-pandemic era, nurses have an incredible opportunity to revitalize theory into practice supporting innovative care practices.

Nursing theory is and calls to be embraced by advanced practice nurses (APNs) as a living tool for care interventions while influencing an equitable health care culture. Nursing theory has aided in transitioning nursing from a vocation to a profession with a unique identity and language and with vast contributions to the practicing nurse. For example, nurses who encounter a patient with a health condition they have minimal experience or knowledge of can look to practice-level nursing theories to lead their nursing care toward patient recovery. Developing knowledge specific to nursing has and will continue to be a driving force for nursing research with successive application to practice. Nursing theory is a thriving concept which began with Florence Nightingale, herself.

The chapter will address the following learning objectives:

1. Recognize the origins of nursing theory.
2. Summarize the evolution of nursing theory's contributions to modern day nursing science.
3. Infer common themes and concepts interwoven through nursing theory exemplars.
4. Distinguish nursing theory as a living tool for APN theory-guided practice.

Historical, Yet Practical Review of the Evolution of Nursing Theory

Florence Nightingale is known as a pioneer for the modern-day nurse. Nightingale elevated the standard of care to emphasize the creation of a safe, clean environment for healing. In doing so, she developed the first nursing theory, environmental theory, which included the principles of healing, leadership, and global action (Riegel et al., 2021). To consider nursing care under these three principles in the mid-1800s during the Crimean War was nothing short of a first in nursing history and placed nursing on the track to evolve into the art and science practiced today.

A major contribution of Nightingale was introducing a philosophy of nursing centralized in holistic nursing care. Nightingale maintained the ideals of critical thinking aimed at providing just care for all. Her later education model would premise nurses to develop clinical decision-making based on holistic thinking no matter the context of practice. Under Nightingale's theory, nursing became the conduit for individuals to prevent disease, recover from illness, and heal from injury. The nurse was present to guide and support the healing journey.

Nightingale rooted an epistemological approach to the nursing discipline. From her work, the nursing metaparadigm (health, person, nursing, and environment) was conceived. The attention to holistic care allowed for the metaparadigm to create a fluid relationship with not only science, but with today's technology while integrating a whole human approach—a relationship that would experience burdens and challenges during the COVID-19 pandemic.

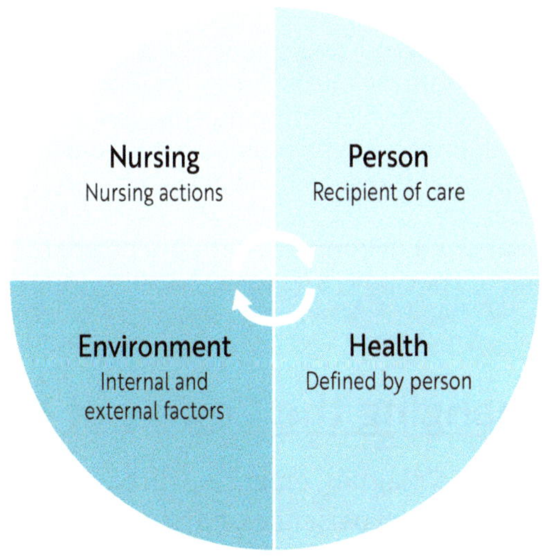

FIGURE 1.1 Nursing metaparadigm.

A fundamental principle of environmental theory relies on a person's maintenance of vital functions to satisfy basic needs in cohesion with the nurse's role (Riegel et al., 2021). At the center of the theory, the environment influences all matters affiliated with life, whereas these influences can either prevent disease or contribute to its proliferation. When applying environmental theory to the COVID-19 pandemic, similarities arise between soldiers on a battlefield more than a century ago to the biological war fought against a microorganism (coronavirus). Nurses from all clinical arenas contributed to key public health initiatives based on the theoretical underpinnings of Nightingale's theory. As prevention and health promotion became the intent of health care messaging during the pandemic, nurses were instrumental in distributing education and knowledge surrounding the mitigation of COVID-19.

These principles laid forth by Nightingale prevail today. Despite the challenges of modern-day nursing to meet patient needs, Nightingale's contribution of holistic critical thinking continues to guide nursing practice. In close analysis of today's health care challenges in a post-pandemic era, a reflection on Nightingale's work reminds us of the vital need to reinvigorate the principles of scientific, ethical, and social commitments to nursing as a science using theory to guide the way.

Florence Nightingale

Birthdate: May 12, 1820

Theory: Environmental theory

Major concept advancing nursing science: Instituted principles used in modern practice of nursing with a focus on individual health and the nurse's role in assessing and creating nursing care aimed at controlling environmental influences. Nightingale created environmental theory through observations and research, heightening nursing's contributions to nursing science.

APN considerations: Environmental theory promotes holistic critical thinking essential to specialty roles for supporting innovative practice.

Theorists Changing the Course of Nursing

As history has presented plagues, emerging diseases, weather events, and unexpected traumatic life experiences, nursing has maintained a consistent presence in healing while guiding others to a return to individualized wellness. How nurses have responded to patient needs has been influenced by nursing theory. Nursing theory provides a foundation of knowledge and related concepts by using a reasonable structure of expectations, hypotheses, and ideas, all of which can be used in a variety of nursing care situations. Theory can be used to further understand the care situation in greater context while inspiring innovative nursing approaches to address individual needs. The APN whether in the role as a clinician, educator, or administrator, can gain foresight into their key functions by using nursing theory in a similar manner. To guide a richer understanding of modern-day nursing, nursing theorists have paved the way to ensure nursing addresses care situations in practical yet holistic methods. Grand theories were first developed by nurse academics to define nursing and structure the nurse's actions (practice), environment, and the professional role of the nurse distinct to the role of the physician. Due to the nature of grand theories being more abstract, they provide nursing with a general framework for practice and can be applied to a wide variety of nursing care situations and environment. An extension of grand nursing theories came in the development of middle-range nursing theories, which grew in development in the 1980s and 1990s, to address phenomenon specific to nursing practice and guide nursing research. The middle-range theory is valuable to students at all academic levels due to providing a middle reality view of generalized practice areas for nurses. Both grand and middle-range theories are purposeful guides and tools for the nurse. A review of Virginia Henderson, Ernestine Wiedenbach, Hildegard Peplau, and Faye Glenn Abdellah will provide a construct of how nursing theory has evolved, threads essential concepts, such as holism, and has contributed to today's nursing theory-guided practice (NTGP) framework.

TABLE 1.1 Comparison of Grand and Middle-Range Nursing Theories' Usability for the Practicing Nurse

Grand Nursing Theory	Major Assumption	Theory's Focus	RN Usability	APN Usability
Dorothea Orem's self-care theory	Successfully meeting universal and development self-care requisites is an important component of primary care prevention and ill health	Addresses individual self-care capacity and suggests ways for its improvement through patient education and other nursing interventions	Guides RNs to prioritize care given a person's situation while promoting individual autonomy through patient education	Guides APNs in promoting self-care ability of each patient encounter, particularly for those individuals who are incapable of adequate health monitoring and making necessary provisions to meet their self-care needs
Middle-Range Nursing Theory	**Major Assumption**	**Theory's Focus**	**RN Usability**	**APN Usability**
Katharine Kolcaba's comfort theory	Human beings react to complex stimuli holistically and that comfort is a desirable holistic outcome	Centered on the identification of patient needs and emphasizes the significance of holistic care	Guides RNs to focus specifically on providing and promoting comfort	Guides APNs to utilize knowledge of holistic care principles while addressing psychological and social factors in human health

Virginia Henderson's Nursing Need Theory

Virginia Henderson contributed a working definition of nursing. Henderson (1978) describes nursing as primarily helping people (sick or well) in the performance of those activities contributing to health, or its recovery (or peaceful death) that they would perform unaided if they had the necessary strength, will, or knowledge and is likewise the unique contribution of nursing to help people to be independent of such assistance as soon as possible. This definition expands nursing's outreach beyond the sick to healthy people and extends beyond care for recovery to sharing knowledge with the end goal for individuals to function independently. A poem by Henderson illustrates the nuances of what is nursing.

> Nursing is temporarily
> the conscious of the unconscious,
> the love of the life of the suicidal
> the leg of the amputee,
> the eyes of the newly blind
> the locomotion of the newborn,
> the knowledge and confidence of the new mother
> and a voice for those too weak to speak (Henderson, 1966)

Virginia Henderson's nursing need theory is a grand theory, but the principles can be applied to many nursing specialties and levels of nursing practice. Henderson's theory focuses on activities associated with living, such as breathing (within normal limits) and sleep/rest. A total of 14 needs are described in Henderson's theory, succeeding the assumption that nursing is an analytical process, hence making need theory applicable to a wider net of health care disciplines. A grounding postulation of nursing need theory is that it is only limited by the imagination and the competence of the nurse who interprets it (Henderson, 2006). Henderson's theory supports nursing to specialize and advance nursing-specific practice roles.

Henderson's theory further explains nursing as an engineer of health by assisting the individual to function independently within their environment. Once again, the critical nature to fully understand the influence of environment on one's health is evident in many nursing theoretical assumptions. The nurse views the environment from the lens of patient safety. Adverse patient outcomes may be the result without the nurse's recognition of patient needs in a supported, safe environment. Even though Henderson does not focus on the environment in her grand theory, it is assumed as an extension of the patient.

From the perspective of the APN, Henderson's need theory can provide a vision of advanced nursing care to focus on enhancing self-efficacy to thrive in one's environment, whether the environment includes a clinical setting, an educational setting, or a leadership setting. Limiting APNs' lens of care to the individual only limits their scope of practice and influence on health and well-being. The restorative underpinnings of Henderson's need theory can be a valuable tool for the APN to address various challenges faced in health care as well as nursing's presence and reaction to these challenges.

Virginia Henderson

Birthdate: November 30, 1897

Theory: Nursing need theory

Major concept advancing nursing science: Henderson developed nursing theory and defined the phenomenon of nursing separate from other health care professions. Henderson positioned the nurse to use judgment based on scientific knowledge to assist individual needs.

APN considerations: The APN can be instrumental in advancing the practice of nursing by emphasizing nursing judgment as unique and contributory in multiple facets of the health care continuum.

Ernestine Wiedenbach's Prescriptive Theory

Ernestine Wiedenbach extended the concept of nursing care to include service to others, stating nursing is a practical phenomenon involving action (Wiedenbach, 1970). Through Wiedenbach' s model, a commitment to quality of health is revealed through the nurse's actions toward the patient. Wiedenbach (1970) further supports nursing by describing four beliefs of human beings that involve dignity, worth, autonomy, and individuality. Wiedenbach postulated that all nurses regardless of specialty gain a personal philosophy regarding dignity, worth, autonomy, and individuality to guide their practice and assist in identifying patient needs. In turn, nursing actions are focused on meeting a central purpose.

A central purpose of nursing is individualized to each nurse, hence strengthening a commitment to care for others. A core attribute of Wiedenbach's theory is to look beyond the recognition that a need exists to be skilled in identifying the need in terms mutually understood by both the

> *"Practice is the what of dynamic nursing, and the focus of practice is the experiencing individual."*
>
> *—Wiedenbach (1962)*

patient and the care provider. APNs are positioned to be instrumental in identifying needs of patients, communities, and colleagues by using the Wiedenbach's theory in action by integrating a keen skill of observation within their role environments. Making assumptions regarding the need for nursing care can result in futile efforts and vacant outcomes; with the active work in observation, ministry (care), and validation (interventions), nursing care can be competent and fruitful for the patient and the APN.

In addition to a central purpose, Wiedenbach's theory consists of prescription and realities.

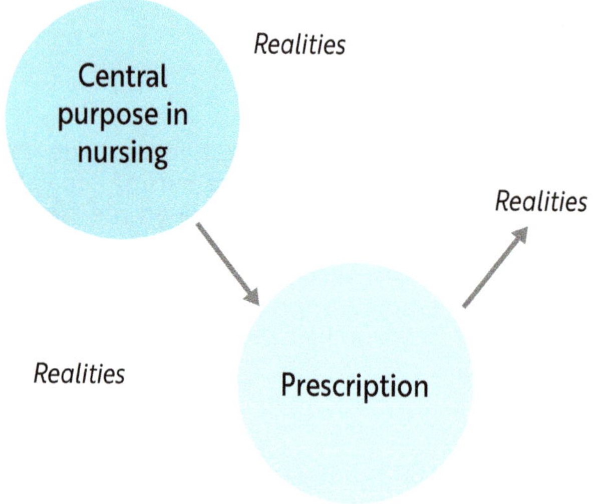

FIGURE 1.2 The helpful art of clinical nursing by Ernestine Wiedenbach.

Under the process for the APN to apply Wiedenbach's prescriptive theory, the prescription constitutes in what manner the APN will address the identified need. Realities are those influencing attributes the patient, community, or colleagues interact with that may impact how the need is first identified and subsequently how effective the prescription is received and carried out. Much of the realities are environmentally based, and the skilled APN understands personal and social influences can confound one's realties as well. Environmental pressures are threaded through many nursing theories and become well-defined concepts for the APN to recognize and evaluate proficiently.

Ernestine Wiedenbach

Birthdate: August 18, 1900

Theory: Prescriptive theory

Major concept advancing nursing science: Wiedenbach expanded the role of the nurse to create her own prescriptive theory in practice by acknowledging the critical steps of a central purpose, a prescription (nursing's clinical judgement), and realities as influential factors.

APN considerations: The APN is a leader in the nursing profession and should elevate their unique roles to differentiate fact from assumption and relate cause to effect in all APN settings.

Hildegard Peplau's Theory of Interpersonal Relations

Historically, nursing care was custodial in nature, and therefore an emphasis on forming a relationship with the patient was not encouraged. Conversely, Hildegard Peplau believed nursing could simply not occur without a relationship between nurse and patient (Peden, 2018). Peplau (1992) described nursing as "a significant, therapeutic, and an interpersonal process" (p. 13). A central theme of Peplau's theory is to promote the forward movement of personality in the direction of a creative, constructive, productive, personal, and community living. As Nightingale introduced the concept of holism, Peplau interwove holism within the nurse-patient relationship by engaging the nurse to further assess the patient's psychological, emotional, and spiritual domains (Peplau, 1991).

To endorse this forward movement, Peplau (1991) organized the theory into three working phases: the orientation phase, the working phase, and the termination phase. Each phase is not intended to be viewed in silo but as overlapping, with the ability to be adjusted based on the nurse's assessment of the clinical situation and the patient's changing needs. Through Peplau's work, nurses are engaged with the individual in a process that promotes respect and sharing knowledge and information and thus delivering an active example of NTGP. APNs can incorporate Peplau's theory into their unique roles by growing in communication skills, continuous evaluation of personal strengths, and a comprehensive understanding of human behavior. The process of communication becomes a critical element within the nurse-patient relationship to encourage and support change in patient behaviors.

Just as Peplau (1991) states, "Nursing is an educative instrument, a maturing force that aims to promote forward movement of (care)" (p. 6), communication becomes a key element to using Peplau's theory in practice.

The exchange of information between the health care provider(s) and the patient is a delicate one, which can be lost in translation for the patient. To further describe Peplau's theoretical assumptions actively used in clinical practice, consider the evolution of bedside reporting. The patient is at the center of two dimensions, the environment and direct communication. The bedside reporting process supports a cultivation of trust, understanding, respect, and satisfaction for the patient.

As the APN cultivates communication skills acquiesced for their unique roles (clinician, educator, and administrator), their work becomes nurse driven with an emphasis on a collaborative approach, building the same characteristics as represented in the example of bedside reporting for the patient. Whether the recipient of the APN's work is a patient, a colleague, staff, or students, using Peplau's theory of interpersonal relations demonstrates holistic communication in fostering connections and working collaboratively toward a mutual goal. Peplau's concept of psychodynamic nursing lays a foundation for the APN to consider personality traits and human behavior trends as contributory to addressing pressing needs or issues. The APN can embody the symbolism of a guide to assist others they interact with in their specialty roles by anticipating reactions and next steps (needs). A caveat of Peplau's theory is the essential task of self-awareness to deal with any biases that may negatively drive deterred assessments. The APN is challenged to view theory through an innovative yet practical lens to not only endorse the growth of the profession, but to engage in effective yet inspiring practice.

Hildegard Peplau

Birthdate: September 1, 1909

Theory: Interpersonal relations theory

Major concept advancing nursing science: The nurse and patient work in partnership to meet mutual goals towards wellness.

APN considerations: The application of Peplau's concept of psychodynamic nursing can contribute to the APN understanding their own behavior and hence reactions to patients, the public, and colleagues. The APN can subsequently choose a therapeutic approach to communication and interpersonal processes integral to creating an efficient and effective care environment.

Faye Glenn Abdellah's 21 Nursing Problems

As an expert in public health, Faye Glenn Abdellah fostered nursing as a science, establishing nursing diagnoses at a time when many did not consider diagnoses part of a nurse's role. From this transition, Abdellah supported nurses as a unique provider of care focused on nursing problems, health, and, poignantly, problem solving. Not only did Abdellah change the course of nursing from disease centered to patient centered, but she also supported the nurse as a problem solver by developing opportunities to meet patient needs in a comprehensive manner.

In Abdellah's 21 nursing problems, the nurse learns to assess patient needs through a 10-step process beginning with learning to know the patient. The process promotes creativity and problem-solving skills to address patient total health needs from immediacy to restoration. The concept of holism is once again threaded into theory as it fosters comprehensive care and continuous assessment. Holism includes the assessment of physical, psychological, and spiritual needs, but in Abdellah's theory it extends beyond the individual to family and social support structures. Environment (as highlighted by Nightingale, Henderson, and Peplau) stands out as a vital factor in steering patient needs. APNs skilled in environmental assessments will undoubtedly be prepared to meet the demands of their specialty roles in today's health care climate.

The 21 nursing problems are intertwined with sociological, physical, and emotional problems through an outcome-based approach. As students learn nursing science and care practices, Abdellah recognized a way to visualize and evaluate competency centered on outcome measures (Abdellah & Levine, 1994). APNs can utilize Abdellah's theory to enhance individual practice by strategizing and structuring interventions. Innovation is a concept in need of further support for the APN and can be highlighted throughout Abdellah's theory by navigating nursing interventions to best support nurse–patient relationships.

Faye Glenn Abdellah

Birthdate: March 13, 1919

Theory: Twenty-one nursing problems

Major concept advancing nursing science: Abdellah developed the system diagnosis-related group among numerous improvements to nursing education. Abdellah provided a conceptual model to identify patient needs through problem analysis. A logical approach to nursing assessment and care approach is central to Abdellah's work, which engaged nursing to use research and logic to problem solve rather than experiential work.

APN considerations: The APN can find support and guidance in Abdellah's work by engaging in nursing research, whether as the active role as researcher or in dissemination of research findings, to deliver innovative solutions (logical and inductive reasoning) to health care challenges.

Timeline of Nursing: An Integration of Nursing Theory Development

The history of nursing has changed philosophically and in practice. From a century ago of informal training to a nursing education system with various scopes of practice, nursing has made a tremendous imprint on caring for the sick and restoring health. Understanding nursing's most influential participants is one small piece to viewing nursing's contributions to care for people yesterday and in the present. An archive of nursing's contributions and professional growth as a science is critical to its present functions and future strategies. Reviewing nursing's timeline beyond dates is a good reminder to all students that nursing is an active discipline devoted to elevating the human experience toward a sense of well-being.

Through a hermeneutic lens, nursing has evolved to redefine itself in many ways. From a service of care to a science of practice, nursing will continue its path toward impacting the health of people through a holistic approach. Nursing's commitment to advocacy, or the act of nurturing, remains central to its purpose and forward movement as leaders in health care. This section will evaluate nursing theory and its impact on how we prepare nurses to practice, use nursing theory as a building block to research, and focus on theory's role as a living tool in a post-pandemic era for the APN.

Overview of Nursing Theory's Impact: From Education to Theory Utilization

Nursing theory's origins are profoundly nestled in academia. The progression of nursing theory was stimulated in the 1950s with an effort to have nursing established as an academic discipline. In 1964, Myrtle Irene Brown (1964) stated, "A clear mandate has been made to nurse researchers to build a body of scientifically tested nursing theory from which may be drawn facts, concepts, and principles on which to base the education of nurses and the nursing care and service of patients, families, and communities" (p. 111). Brown's declaration was clear. Nursing began to establish research questions underpinned by nursing theories; hence nursing would create new knowledge specific to nursing science.

To provide historical context, after WWII, nursing engaged in ongoing efforts to be a distinct voice among health care disciplines. The efforts of nurse scholars exemplified this desire for nursing to have autonomy by investing in research focused on patient care in alignment to the time's public health needs and advances of medical science. Surgical and medical innovations, such as open-heart surgery and kidney dialysis, were making major impacts on the patient care continuum (illness to recovery). Nursing has an innate conscience of patient care, transcending the understanding to grow as a distinct discipline by advancing nursing knowledge (science) as an integral component to the role of the nurse (caregiver). Nursing would begin its progression to a systematic science by adhering to a process of observation, research, and ultimately evidence-based practice (EBP). Nurse researchers would invest in scientific inquiry to guide practice rather than intuition to meet the growing demands of patient care.

In 1963, the Surgeon General's Consultant Group on Nursing (1963) called for support of nursing research to focus on "patient-oriented studies in line with the changing patterns of nursing care" (p. 55). One year later, Virginia Henderson (1964) published an article, "The Nature of Nursing," calling for research to focus on clinical nursing to secure nursing as an independent professional practice. This was a historical turning point for nursing research and nursing theory. Prior to the 1960s, most nursing research was aimed at education of nursing practice and retention of the nursing workforce. A quote from Dorothy Johnson (1959) capitulates this change:

> The question of the existence of a body of substantive knowledge which can be called the science of nursing ... is a question of considerable significance for nursing's continued development as a recognized professional discipline. Certainly, no profession can long exist without making explicit its theoretical bases for practice so that this knowledge can be communicated, tested, and expanded. (p. 291)

During this evolution of nursing research, nursing education was also under major changes. Nursing programs were extending from hospital schools to colleges and universities, offering varying pathways to enter nursing practice. A lag in fully embracing the need for nursing research to focus on practice was evident in the academic setting and would take longer to engage nurses with advanced degree preparations to focus on practice-based research. A reaction to this need inspired the establishment of nursing doctoral programs. Concurrently, there was an ongoing need of nurse recruitment. Nursing would find challenges in the next 2 decades to recruit in the profession and diversify its workforce. Despite the understood need to advance nursing science and establish itself as a distinct health care profession, nursing academia would struggle to legitimize nursing theory as a construct tethering science to practice.

During the 1970s medicine did not use theory to ground its research, which questioned nursing's attempt to use theory to underpin its scientific growth. In reflection of historical context, nursing began its journey to legitimization in the 1950s and 1960s, when many nurse academics used the social and behavioral sciences as models to guide their research efforts.

Social and behavioral sciences use theory to develop knowledge specific to their specialties. Nursing postulated the use of nursing theory would afford a required boundary to separate itself from biomedical disciplines. As the evolution of nursing as a science would continue, it became evident that to meet the demands of the fast-paced innovations impacting the medical care of patients, nursing would need to focus on building practice theories to address situation-specific patient needs. With attention on growing nursing science, the nursing metaparadigm was reinvigorated. As nursing has strived to care for the whole person, its research efforts would attempt to do the same by directing empirical research through four major themes: person, environment, health, and nursing. The sentiment is best portrayed by Fawcett (1980), who described "persons as biopsychosocial beings in constant interaction with and influenced by their social and physical environments" (p. 11). With the core philosophy of nursing remaining on the care of individual from illness to recovery, nursing theory would expand as a grounding framework for care in action.

Emphasis of Theory as a Building Block to Nursing Research

A reflection on what nursing theory is assists students and APNs to formulate perceptions regarding NTGP. Brown (1964) suggests nursing theory should provide the foundations of nursing practice, help to generate further knowledge, and indicate which direction nursing should develop in the future. According to Chinn and Jacobs (1978), nursing theory aims to describe, predict, and explain the phenomenon of nursing. Nursing theory provides the principles underpinning practice (Colley, 2003, p. 33). As APNs practice in different roles (clinician, educator, and administrator), nursing theory becomes a valuable tool to assist in the changing landscape of health care, beginning with nursing research.

Health care is a dynamic and fragile environment. Challenges are a constant urging for flexible solutions while maintaining the patient at the center of care. Nursing has answered the call with reciprocal flexibility by using scientific inquiry and empiric support for evidence-based nursing care. It is through the advances of nursing science, nursing research has stimulated a body of knowledge and a lexis for other health care disciplines to look to nursing for innovative solutions to some of the more perplexing health care challenges, much like those experienced through the COVID-19 pandemic. To make change necessitates a theoretical perspective and a direction toward scientific inquiry.

According to Hickman (2019), "Nursing theory and science are open, dynamic systems" (p. 85). Considering the concept of an open, dynamic system, change becomes a defining attribute. As health care emerges from the COVID-19 pandemic, APNs are positioned to be leaders in change by employing rigorous scientific inquiry to make a positive impact on how health care is delivered and accepted by people worldwide. Nonetheless, a keystone to this change is grounded in nursing theory to support the valued and incalculable use of evidence-based nursing care. Nursing theory engages thinking like a nurse through the viewpoint of a nurse. With nursing theory and a nursing philosophy to guide research, nursing endures as a discipline committed to care of the person.

Nursing theory has been germane to nursing science as an underpinning of practice. To illustrate, the American Association of Colleges of Nursing (AACN, 2006) includes nursing theory in the DNP (Doctor of Nursing Practice) essentials document under essential. DNP-prepared APNs are expected to have the ability to translate knowledge swiftly and effectively to benefit patients within the daily demands of all types of practice environments. The AACN has called for DNP-prepared APNs to develop and evaluate new practice approaches based on nursing theories as well as theories from other disciplines.

In addition, the AACN (2010) asserts the PhD requires "a strong scientific emphasis within the discipline; an understanding of science in related disciplines and translational science" (p. 2), and in preparing a "steward of the discipline," the PhD curriculum needs to include "theoretical/scientific underpinnings of nursing and other disciplines" (p. 5). The importance of nursing theory lies in its ability to direct research through a nursing lens, therefore supporting and adding to a body of distinct nursing knowledge. For the APN, acknowledgement of the relationship between theory and research is one that is interrelated. In other words, theory guides research, and research informs theory (Patterson, 2021, p. 337):

> Although the investigator may not have been thinking of theory explicitly when he or she developed the research question or selected the intervention, theoretical thinking is the foundation to planning and implementing all meaningful research. (Day, 2017, p. 13)

An Introduction of Reorganizing Theory for the Post-Pandemic Era

Evidence has been offered to support nursing theory as a cornerstone to nursing as a discipline with a distinct body of knowledge. The value of theory as a practical tool to support innovative change needs to be obtainable to APNs. As much as the pandemic overwhelmed health care systems, nurses were consistent in their presence and response to a demanding environment. The impact of COVID-19's disruption of standard care protocols forcing nurses to quickly adapt is not lost to most nurse educators and leaders. Despite the hardships experienced by health care providers, the pandemic highlighted opportunity. Opportunities for change were present not just from necessity, but from a position of innovation. Current trends in innovation in health care include areas within education, technology, and a changing workforce. All three areas are pathways for the APN to consider within their specialty roles of educator, clinician, and administrator (leader).

Nursing became a valued contributor as part of a multidisciplinary approach to COVID-19. Nurses were engaged in roles associated with infection control, team-based patient care, and health surveillance due to the temporary removal of barriers from federal and state policymakers. A summation of RNs' contributions during the pandemic is eloquently stated by Schwerdtle et al. (2020), who describes nurses as "thought leaders, operational innovators, and trusted partners." Nurses and APNs have been in a paradigm shift since the beginning of the pandemic, decreasing barriers to change. With this decrease in barriers arises an opportunity to reorganize nursing theory as a practical tool to ensure nursing's voice is embedded and leading change in health care delivery.

Nursing education has an equally vital responsibility to cultivate a growing curiosity for innovation among students to address care practice challenges and lead the path to a more responsive and holistic health care environment. As part of the impact of the pandemic, many nursing education programs adjusted to virtual platforms. Whether the educational program was prelicensure, master's, or doctoral, the changes were abrupt. Concepts such as digital literacy, e-learning, and flexible learning became core topics of discussion and ongoing evaluations. For some students, the transition was welcomed, and for others the distance created a divide in their learning process, with subsequent effects on progression in/into the nursing profession. Pedagogy and modes of educational delivery were transformed as abruptly as caring for a patient. The remote platforms of learning were viewed as an emergency response, but the technology of remote learning became increasingly embraced by nurse educators to fulfill already limited clinical placements and enhance a fluid succession of educational learning objectives. The growing popularity of digital learning has led many nursing programs to offer online options; however, the demand for quality nursing education is needed more than ever. Since the pandemic, public health has rapidly changed, with a greater need to address populations in which nurses serve. Social determinants of health (SDOH) and health equity are enduring critical elements to integrate into nursing curricula. Nursing theory, as a philosophical underpinning to nursing education, can offer opportunities to strengthen nursing educational programs to better educate future nurses and nurse leaders.

As adjustments were quickly made to utilize technology as a solution to meet patient needs, it became more apparent technology is a mainstay to health care delivery. Telehealth (telecommunication), remote monitoring, and wearable health devices were vastly used to stay abreast of patient needs when the people were physically distant from one another. Predictive analytics and diagnostic algorithms expanded health care providers' ability to provide care. As many of these technologies offered emergent solutions, nursing understood the obligation the profession had to treat the whole person (physical, psychological, and spiritual). Many nurses struggled with an ethical commitment to care in a holistic manner during the pandemic. Despite technology remaining a constant and ever-changing element to health care, nurses and APNs can embrace technology through the principles of many nursing theories. By highlighting and aligning nursing theory to the utilization of technology in nursing practice, nurses can address this ethical dilemma and ensure technology meets the needs of the whole patient.

A healthy workforce is essential to adapting to change and fostering innovation. Since the pandemic, the nursing workforce has changed significantly. Gaps exist in the nursing workforce as a result of the burdens placed on nurses during the pandemic, exposing a threat to nurses' financial, psychological, and physical resilience (National Academies of Sciences, Engineering, and Medicine et al., 2021). According to the National Academies of Sciences, Engineering, and Medicine et al. (2021), the nursing workforce is challenged to meet the growing health care needs of the population nurses serve while increasing its own diversity. APNs can meet these demands by encouraging growth and knowledge of nursing theory to address a need for a more diversified nursing workforce. The post-pandemic era is a unique period for APNs to carry the momentum of innovation and use nursing theory as a foundation to expand nursing knowledge and the nursing workforce while enhancing nursing care and leadership practices.

Theory Guiding APN Practice: A Case Study Examination

To enhance understanding and application of nursing theory to the role of the APN, case studies are provided throughout the book to assist the student in valuable practice reflection and critical thinking to align common practice scenarios to nursing theory. The goal of the provided case studies is to energize and inform the APN student to select, evaluate, and innovate practice through nursing theory. The following case study is an example of the case studies provided in each chapter.

Case Study I

Applying Virginia Henderson's Need Theory to APN Practice Roles

Scenario

The patient, Ms. Y, is a female 22-year-old college student working part-time as a waitress while attending school full-time to become an accountant. Ms. Y is being seen at a student health clinic with thoughts of suicide and self-harm. Upon further examination, Ms. Y is transported to the closest community hospital due to episodes of vomiting in the clinic and acute change in mental status with a report from Ms. Y's roommate that she ingested toilet cleaner.

Ms. Y is admitted to the medical unit. Her present physical assessment reveals she is alert and oriented, and a CT scan and endoscopy revealed damage to the larynx, mouth, with stomach ulcers present. Ms. Y displays signs of depression and withdraws from speaking to the health care team. She is resisting oral fluid intake.

Ms. Y's mother is present and reports her daughter has been depressed for about 6 months since her break-up with a long-term boyfriend of 3 years.

Henderson's Need Theory/Major Assumptions

- Increase patient independence through nursing activities based on 14 human needs.
    - The first nine components are physiological. The 10th and 14th are psychological aspects of communicating and learning. The 11th component is spiritual and moral. The 12th and 13th components are sociologically oriented to occupation and recreation (Meleis, 2007).
- The nurse's roles include a substitutive role (doing for the person), a supplementary role (helping the person), and a complimentary role (working with the person).
- Focus is on individual care.
- Patients should be assisted by nurses to maintain health, recover from illness, or achieve a peaceful death.

Henderson's 14 Needs **Physiologic (P)** **Psychologic (PY)** **Spiritual (S)** **Sociologic (SO)**	**Patient Assessment**	**APN Theory-Supported Intervention** **Clinician (C)**	**APN Theory-Supported Intervention** **Management/ Leadership (ML)**	**APN Theory-Supported Intervention** **Educator (E)**
1. Breathe normally (P)	Ms. Y RR 24: Irregular with O2 saturation of 93% on room air	(C) Observe for signs of harming self while assessing for activity intolerance related to dyspnea and periods of hyperventilation	(ML) Ensure in rounding that patient's needs are being heard and assess all potential available resources within the health care system	(E) Educate staff/ students on S/S of anxiety (hyperventilation) and physical and psychological effects of depression

Henderson's 14 Needs **Physiologic (P)** **Psychologic (PY)** **Spiritual (S)** **Sociologic (SO)**	**Patient Assessment**	**APN Theory-Supported Intervention** **Clinician (C)**	**APN Theory-Supported Intervention** **Management/ Leadership (ML)**	**APN Theory-Supported Intervention** **Educator (E)**
2. Nutrition (P)	Ms. Y is 5 ft. 4 in. and weighs 55 kg. Skin turgor is normal, no tenting; refuses to drink any liquid despite a prescribed liquid diet post–toilet cleaner ingestion; lips are dry and cracked	(C) Observe for signs of anxiety and all other sources of stressors contributing to activity intolerance and mental/social health; build a therapeutic patient–practitioner relationship	(ML) Ensure interdisciplinary collaboration is supported between dietary and nutritionist, providers, and nursing staff	(E) Educate staff/ students on importance of hydration and S/S of dehydration leading to activity intolerance amid energy expenditures with physical manifestations of depression
3. Elimination (P)	Minimal urine output reported by nursing staff since admission	(C) Prescribe Foley catheter placement to monitor hydration status and labs to assess for renal function	(ML) Ensure policies and procedures are in place and readily available to staff regarding evidence-based placement and monitoring of Foley catheter to avoid risk for infection	(E) Educate staff/ students on purpose and procedure of Foley catheter
4. Movement and posturing (P)	Ms. Y complains of fatigue and is unable to get out of bed with observed gait imbalance	(C) Prescribe out of bed as tolerated with assistance; continue to build therapeutic relationship to encourage activity tolerance	(ML) Ensure policies and procedures are in place and readily available to staff regarding falls risk	(E) Educate staff/ students on assessment of falls risk and therapeutic communication to support increase in activity tolerance

Henderson's 14 Needs Physiologic (P) Psychologic (PY) Spiritual (S) Sociologic (SO)	Patient Assessment	APN Theory-Supported Intervention Clinician (C)	APN Theory-Supported Intervention Management/ Leadership (ML)	APN Theory-Supported Intervention Educator (E)
5. Sleep and rest (P)	Ms. Y has experienced less than 2 to 3 hours of sleep for the last 10 days with observable signs of exhaustion, including complaints of frequent headaches, heart palpitations, and joint pain	(C) Prescribe EKG to rule out heart dysrhythmias, Tylenol PM for pain, and continue to provide therapeutic communication to assist patient to recovery and independence	(ML) Ensure unit promotes quiet, rest time for patients while supporting staff in efficient work processes and environment	(E) Educate staff/students on assessment of exhaustion and physical as well as mental complications from lack of rest/ sleep
6. Suitable clothing (P)	Ms. Y was admitted wearing a loose-fitting dress and had unclean hair and dirt under fingernails	(C) Assess for patient willingness to bathe and complete/ perform personal hygiene as signs of recovery; use empathetic communication	(ML) Ensure staff provide time to assist patient in completing personal hygiene with available bathing products; have an accessible procedure for staff to ensure patient privacy and safety while performing self-care	(E) Educate staff/ students on assessment of signs and symptoms of depression/ exhaustion and apply evidence-based nursing interventions to comfort the patient while supporting the patient toward independence
7. Maintain body temperature (P)	Ms. Y has no signs of hypo- or hyperthermia	(C) Assess for change in patient status to indicate signs and symptoms of infection	(ML) Ensure staff remains abreast of unit policies and procedures regarding risk for infection among various patient populations	(E) Educate staff/ students on risk for infection related to decrease in activity and invasive procedures

Henderson's 14 Needs Physiologic (P) Psychologic (PY) Spiritual (S) Sociologic (SO)	Patient Assessment	APN Theory-Supported Intervention Clinician (C)	APN Theory-Supported Intervention Management/ Leadership (ML)	APN Theory-Supported Intervention Educator (E)
8. Keep body cleaned and well groomed (P)	Ms. Y's mother reports that previous to the last couple months her daughter was very conscientious of appearance and was well groomed	(C) Assess for improvement in body hygiene with referrals to mental health consults	(ML) Ensure staff appropriately report/chart changes in patient appearance to providers on an interdisciplinary level	(E) Educate staff/ students on S/S of depression and effects of poor hygiene on overall health and wellness
9. Avoid dangers in the environment (P)	Evidence of attempt of suicide; notable S/S of depression and exhaustion with risk of dehydration and malnutrition; poor gait	(C) Ongoing assessment of risk of harm with employed referrals for mental health evaluation and resources; continue to create therapeutic relationship with patient to support progression to independence	(ML) Ensure staff is competent in assessing patient environment for potential items to harm self with removal of items to create a safe patient environment; ensure policies are in place and accessible to staff on risk for self-harm	(E) Educate staff/ students on risk of environmental dangers with a patient at increased risk for self-harm and other safety concerns, such as falls and mental acuity due to less than adequate liquid and caloric intake
10. Communication (PY)	Damage noted to larynx as a result of toilet cleaner ingestion; has hoarse speech	(C) Assess for improvement to speech while encouraging communication in a therapeutic relationship	(ML) Ensure adequate staffing to meet unit patient acuity, including time to assess for patient needs	(E) Educate staff/ students on employing effective and clear communication to patients with impaired verbal communication

Henderson's 14 Needs Physiologic (P) Psychologic (PY) Spiritual (S) Sociologic (SO)	Patient Assessment	APN Theory-Supported Intervention Clinician (C)	APN Theory-Supported Intervention Management/ Leadership (ML)	APN Theory-Supported Intervention Educator (E)
11. Worship according to one's faith (S)	Religion: Methodist; Ms. Y's mother reports daughter was active in church choir and assisted in youth group church activities	(C) Assist patient in connecting with spiritual resources in the hospital setting and seek patient needs for spiritual support	(ML) Promote spiritual resource availability to staff to share with patient requests and maintain a culture within the work environment that addresses patient spiritual needs	(E) Educate staff/ students on value of spiritual assessment and inclusion to holistic care practices
12. Work accomplishment (SO)	Ms. Y's mother reports daughter struggling with current course work in college	(C) Continue to build a therapeutic patient relationship and work with other disciplines to engage patient in discussing coping and stress management techniques	(ML) Ensure work environment is supportive to staff to practice in a holistic manner, assessing with a biopsychosocial framework	(E) Educate staff/ students on practicing with a biopsychosocial framework
13. Recreation (SO)	Decrease in self-care; withdrawn from social groups and activities and family events	(C) Continue to build a therapeutic patient relationship and work with other disciplines to engage patient in discussing coping and stress management techniques	(ML) Ensure work environment is supportive to staff to practice in a holistic manner, assessing with a biopsychosocial framework	(E) Educate staff/ students on practicing with a biopsychosocial framework

Henderson's 14 Needs **Physiologic (P)** **Psychologic (PY)** **Spiritual (S)** **Sociologic (SO)**	**Patient Assessment**	**APN Theory-Supported Intervention** **Clinician (C)**	**APN Theory-Supported Intervention** **Management/ Leadership (ML)**	**APN Theory-Supported Intervention** **Educator (E)**
14. Learning (P, PY, SO)	Ms. Y has physical and psychosocial signs of inability to cope with stressors and present illness (depression and effects of toxic substance ingestion)	(C) Provide support to family and patient to address stressors and coping mechanisms	(ML) Ensure work environment is supportive to staff to practice in a holistic manner, assessing with a biopsychosocial framework	(E) Educate staff/ students on assessing and applying care interventions with a biopsychosocial framework

Figure Credits

Fig. 1.1: CJT Consulting & Education, "Nursing Metaparadigm Concepts," https://i0.wp.com/nursingeducationexpert.com/wp-content/uploads/2017/10/NrsgMetaparadigm.png?fit=1334%2C967&ssl=1. Copyright © 2017 by CJT Consulting & Education.

Fig. 1.2: Ernestine Wiedenbach, "Prescriptive Theory," https://www.currentnursing.com/nursing_theory/Ernestine_Wiedenbach.html. Copyright © 2017 by Current Nursing.

CHAPTER 2

A Pillar of the Profession

Key Terms

Carper's patterns of knowing: A theory that describes the different ways nurses gain knowledge. There are four main patterns: empirical, personal, ethical, and aesthetic.

Pedagogy: The study of teaching methods, including the aims of education and the ways in which such goals may be achieved.

National Council Licensure Examination (NCLEX): One of the two standardized tests nurses need to pass in order to become either a licensed practical nurse (LPN) or a registered nurse (RN).

National Council of State Boards of Nursing (NCSBN): A not-for-profit organization whose U.S. members include the nursing regulatory bodies in the 50 states, the District of Columbia, and four U.S. territories.

Associate degree in nursing (ADN): A 2-year degree and the minimum amount of school required to become licensed as an RN. Once the student graduates, they are eligible to take the NCLEX, which must be passed to become licensed by the state. An RN must be licensed to be able to work.

Bachelor of Science in Nursing (BSN): An undergraduate-level degree for RNs that introduces nurses to topics such as patient care technology, research, health promotion, safety, and quality within the health care system.

Master of Science in Nursing (MSN): An advanced-level postgraduate degree for RNs and considered an entry-level degree for nurse educators and managers. The degree also may prepare a nurse to seek a career as a nurse administrator, health policy expert, or clinical nurse leader.

Doctor of Nursing Practice (DNP): The terminal degree in nursing practice. RNs who have earned their DNP can serve as executives, educators, or researchers and provide care for patients with the largest scope of practice available to nurses.

Doctor of Philosophy in Nursing (PhD): A research degree designed to prepare nurse scholars to advance the art, science, and practice of the discipline.

Introduction

Since establishing nursing theory as pinnacle to nursing's identity and its supportive role through practice and research, nursing theories provide a foundation of knowledge to guide actions at all levels of practice and specialties. Nursing theory has been widely accepted as a mainstay to nursing's placement in health care and is integral to its growth as an influential health care profession. Levine (1995) described nursing theory as the intellectual life of nursing in nursing curricula. Over the last few decades, nursing curricula has strived to use theory-related content in curricula at all levels of nursing education. An exploration of nursing theory's presence in nursing programs will support theory's essential nature to prepare students for various levels of nursing practice.

The chapter will address the following learning objectives:

1. Appraise theory's role in nursing knowledge with an analysis of how nurses know what nurses know.
2. Summarize the role of nursing theory in the curricular preparation of diploma graduate nurses.
3. Summarize the role of nursing theory in the curricular preparation of associate degree graduate nurses.
4. Summarize the role of nursing theory in the curricular preparation of baccalaureate graduate nurses.
5. Summarize the role of nursing theory in the curricular preparation of master's-prepared graduate nurses.
6. Summarize the role of nursing theory in the curricular preparation of doctoral-prepared graduate nurses.

Theory and Its Influence on All Levels of Nursing Practice

As nursing theory is a primary factor influencing practice, there remains a lack of recognition for its influence in socializing the student to the role of the nurse and transitioning the nurse to advanced practice roles.

Part of this missed opportunity for theory's recognition is a deficiency of open dialogue in how nurses know what nurses know. In other words, where does nursing knowledge come from, and how do nurses create a knowledge repository for individual practice? Nursing theory helped to answer this question.

In 1978 Barbara Carper developed patterns of knowing theory, premised on the belief that discovery of self and others comes with reflection, synthesis of perception, and connecting to existing knowledge. Over time, it became one of the most influential early nursing theoretical papers (Chinn & Kramer, 2018). According to Carper (1978), nursing knowledge evolution is related to four patterns of knowing: empirical (verifiable observation; factual), aesthetic (art), ethical (principles; morals), and personal (individual). The nurse is committed to an engaged process of learning, whether during structured educational experiences or through active reflection during the act of practicing within the nurse's role. The assumption of Carper's theory engages nurse educators to consider all ways nurses and students learn based on how nursing is perceived and defined. Nursing knowledge is more than learning through a single pathway of science, but rather multifactorial, with a focus on broadening a humanistic aspect of exceptional nursing practice.

Carper's theory inspired educators to approach nursing curricula through creativity, dialogue, and a greater appreciation of individual critical thought. From this inspiration, nursing curricula across all levels of entry (diploma to baccalaureate) and levels of practice (master's and doctoral) have adjusted program philosophies, schematics, and pedagogical approaches to prepare students and nurses to successfully enter practice prepared to meet current challenges in health care. Entry- and graduate-level programs of nursing have changed significantly to meet the demands for nursing and to offer more value-based education in a shorter timeframe. The post-pandemic era is no exception to challenging nursing education's trajectory to ensure nurses and students are prepared to act safely, holistically, and within a nursing framework supported by nursing theory. A guided look at nursing theory's impact at each level of academic preparation will assist the student in cognitively embracing nursing theory as essential to preparing for their role as indispensable contributors of exceptional health care delivery.

> *"It is the general conception of any field of inquiry that ultimately determines the kind of knowledge that field aims to develop as well as the manner in which that knowledge is to be organized, tested, and applied. Such an understanding involves critical attention to the question of what it means to know and what kinds of knowledge are held to be the most value in the discipline of nursing." (Carper, 1978, p.13)*

Reflective Activity

- Complete Examples in Practice column, with reflective consideration of each pattern of knowing for the APN roles of clinician, nurse leader, and nurse educator.

Patterns of Knowing for the APN/Clinician

Pattern of Knowing	Description/Qualities	Examples in Practice
Empirics	Evidence-based nursing · Factual · Objective	
Aesthetics	Art of clinical practice · Empathetic · Subjective · Visionary	
Personal	Relationship-based nursing · Active listening · Authenticity · Empowering · Mutual respect	
Ethics	Principled-based nursing · Standards · Values · Morality	

Patterns of Knowing for the APN/Nurse Leader

Pattern of Knowing	Description/Qualities	Examples in Practice
Empirics	Evidence-based nursing · Factual · Objective	
Aesthetics	Art of clinical practice · Empathetic · Subjective · Visionary	
Personal	Relationship-Based nursing · Active listening · Authenticity · Empowering · Mutual respect	
Ethics	Principled-based nursing · Standards · Values · Morality	

Patterns of Knowing for the APN/Nurse Educator

Pattern of Knowing	Description/Qualities	Examples in Practice
Empirics	Evidence-based nursing • Factual • Objective	
Aesthetics	Art of clinical practice • Empathetic • Subjective • Visionary	
Personal	Relationship-based nursing • Active listening • Authenticity • Empowering • Mutual respect	
Ethics	Principled-based nursing • Standards • Values • Morality	

Pathways to Nursing: Theory's Role

Pathways to nursing vary and speak to the unique needs of traditional and nontraditional students. The nursing shortage has made its imprint on health care delivery. According to the World Health Statistics Report, 3.9 million nurses in the United States do not meet the country's health care needs, and an additional 1 million nurses were projected to be needed in 2020 (Slattery et al., 2016). Not only has this anticipated need placed a burden on health care and nurse sustainability, COVID-19 emerged in early 2020, leading to heightened nursing demands, with subsequent nurses leaving bedside care or the profession. The necessity for nursing programs at all levels of preparation to produce candidates to legally practice is imminent and pressing for many health care systems across the country. Despite the need for nurses, nursing curricula must ensure nursing theory guides educational preparations so that nurses can be prepared to meet the complex demands of health care and the critical needs of patients. The following text will guide you in understanding the role nursing theory has on both the educational preparation and the role of nurses at varying levels of practice.

Diploma-Prepared Nurse

Diploma programs are the oldest education form in preparing students to enter the profession and sit for national examination to be licensed as an

RN. The National Council Licensure Examination, otherwise referred to as NCLEX, is developed psychometrically by the National Council of State Boards of Nursing (NCSBN). Typically, diploma programs are 2 to 3 years and are medical setting based. The diploma program has seen quite the evolution, with its origins as in-house training where students lived or adjacent to hospitals and with the focus of student nurse preparation on apprentice-based learning. Today, diploma programs offer a robust education in social science and biology with an emphasis on clinical learning. Graduates are prepared to find employment in acute care, long-term, and community-based settings and hold strong clinical skills. Currently, there are less than 100 diploma programs in the United States.

Diploma program curriculum offers prerequisite courses often through an affiliation with a local university or college. Nursing specific courses include pharmacology, elements of patient care, and introductions to patient care specialties, such as pediatrics, psychiatric, and acute and chronic care. Due to changes in the NCLEX, nursing programs at large have revised or rewritten program curricula to reflect the examination to better prepare students for safe entry to practice and exam success. Diploma programs are no exception. Curricula changes have evolved to offer conceptual learning, such as care of the patient across the life span and integrate a philosophy-guided curriculum. Oftentimes, a nursing theory framework is embedded into curricula development. Due to shorter length of program and limits to credit hours, students in diploma programs may not be taught a specific nursing theory course; however, a theory is often interwoven throughout the curricula.

A natural alignment of nursing theory to diploma curricula is Virginia Henderson's need theory. Henderson's theory focuses on 14 needs of a patient, ranging from physiological (breathing, eating, elimination), psychological (communication, learning, coping), spiritual (faith, worship, values), and social needs (sense of accomplishment and recreation). The key principle of need theory is to increase patient independence from illness to recovery. Nurse educators can effectively utilize Henderson's need theory within diploma curricula to teach students to create practical therapeutic assessment and interventions to supplement patient needs while supporting the patient on caring for self.

Associate's-Prepared Nurse

The associate degree programs of nursing have remained popular for many years. The associate's nursing programs typically are a 2- to 3-year program with multiple curriculum track options for which graduates earn an associate degree in nursing (ADN). A skills-centered curriculum is the focus of ADN programs; however, many programs offer liberal arts courses as well. A strong emphasis is placed on patient bedside care in that clinicals are key to achieving program outcomes. The National Organization for associate degree Nursing (NOADN) is a professional organization that supports and promotes the associate degree level of entry into nursing. An expectation for graduates of ADN programs is to enter the nursing field with strong clinical skills and as a steppingstone to a bachelor's degree. A common goal for the ADN nurse is to enter the field in a shorter timeframe as an RN, with the potential to earn a bachelor's degree with financial aid from an employer.

The ADN program is enticing, with multiple entry points and curricular pathways, hence reaching a wider range of potential students to prepare (much needed) future nurses. A traditional ADN curriculum provides a daytime traditional track in that students often complete the program in five semesters. A weekend ADN curriculum offers students to earn an associate degree in nursing on weekends with completion in seven semesters. An LPN (licensed practical nurse) to ADN curriculum provides an opportunity for LPNs to enter the program with benefits, resulting in less time than a traditional ADN curriculum with completion in four semesters. The variety of curricular pathways offer an opportunity to educators to integrate and develop curriculum to support nursing knowledge through nursing theory.

Often, nursing theory in ADN programs is viewed through the metaparadigm (person, environment, health, and nursing). As nursing interventions are a primary focus in ADN curricula, the metaparadigm offers an organizing framework to provide students a way to view nursing's role in society and apply the nursing process. In the ADN curricula, theory becomes more prominent to support nursing interventions through research evidence. A major outcome of ADN curricula is to prepare graduates to assist in identifying research problems, assist in data collection, and use research findings in practice.

Baccalaureate-Prepared Nurse

The baccalaureate nursing programs offer traditional and nontraditional tracks or points of entry. A Bachelor of Science Nursing degree (BSN) is offered through colleges or universities with traditional pathways over 4 years and nontraditional pathways ranging from accelerated programs between 18 months and 3 years depending on fulfillment of general education requirements. A draw for many potential students to earn a bachelor's degree in nursing is an increase in average pay per year as well as leadership opportunities in management and advancement in clinical specializations.

Many diploma and ADN graduates return to earn their BSN by completing an RN-BSN pathway, which can be done in 2 or less years. With the growing shortage of RNs, colleges and universities have sought to answer this need by investing into accelerated BSN programs. The accelerated BSN program is unique in that students who have already earned a bachelor's degree in another field of study take additional coursework and clinical work to become a BSN-prepared nurse. Often, accelerated BSN programs can be offered online and have yielded high attrition rates with success on the NCLEX exam.

A distinction with the baccalaureate program is students become acquainted with nursing theory by a separate theory course or though integration throughout the curriculum. A major goal of theory's foundation to the BSN curricula is to assist the student to describe and define the metaparadigm, not only though concepts but also in relationship to other specific nursing concepts. Students are offered curricula that requires critical thinking to make connections and identify relationships to specific nursing theories/theorists. As a result, students are expected to think like a nurse and use theorist-based interventions on individuals and groups with a focus on health promotion and disease prevention.

In addition to the strong theoretical foundation organized in the BSN curriculum, students are directed to critique nursing research by identifying researchable clinical problems/issues, analyzing data collection methods, and applying critical reasoning on how to apply and disseminate research findings to clinical practice. The BSN graduate is educated to understand the practice to theory to research cycle and be engaged in its active process. Through the BSN curricula, the nurse is prepared to collaborate, appraise findings for clinical relevance, and generate a supportive research environment. Theory is placed in a foundational role for the BSN nurse to instill a level of competence and skill, promoting clinical care based on metatheoretical concepts.

Master's-Prepared Nurse

The master's-prepared nurse, or student who has earned a Master of Science in Nursing (MSN), has become more common and a goal for many BSN nurses due to opportunities to engage in nonclinical pathways, such as management and education, and earn advanced practice nursing degrees, such as certified nurse practitioner and certified nurse midwife. Due to the nature of the MSN degree being an endeavor for the adult student, flexible pathways have been developed by colleges and universities. Pathways include but are not limited to an MSN generalist, MSN nurse practitioner (family, acute care, geriatric care, and psychiatric mental health), and MSN nurse administrator.

As the RN decides on an advanced nursing career path, the MSN curriculum, regardless of specialty, prepares nurses to not only understand the practice to theory to research cycle, but to visualize the goal of the research as theory development or theory testing. The MSN-prepared nurse is educated to be engaged in how nursing theory guides nursing research. A critical component to the MSN curriculum across all pathways is the emphasis on reflection, analysis, and critique of nursing theory-guided interventions with theorist-specific evaluation of interventions. Courses within MSN curricula guide students to experiment with and evaluate the utility of different nursing theories. At the MSN level, students are expected to use nursing theories as conceptual frameworks to assess and level the complexity of individual and group needs. MSN-prepared nurses will actively engage in identifying clinical and nonclinical issues related to nursing and seeking to direct the research experience toward replication.

Doctoral-Prepared Nurse

Nurses in doctoral programs, either DNP or PhD, are engaged in using nursing theories to design studies and generate new nursing knowledge. Often students seeking a doctoral degree in nursing choose between the Doctor of Nursing Practice (DNP) or the Doctor of Philosophy in Nursing (PhD). The focus in regard to utilization of nursing theory remains the same for both doctoral-prepared nurses to advance nursing science. A distinction lies in the specifics and breadth of research explored. The DNP nurse may focus on translating research to practice while improving patient outcomes and dissemination of nursing knowledge. The PhD nurse may focus on the testing and development of theory within the domains of health care and social, economic, political, and ethical issues important to nursing.

Doctoral-prepared nurses are pivotal in explaining the practice to theory to research cycle through continuous expansion of nursing science to provide a source for nursing-specific interventions. Doctoral students are provided curricula that demonstrates how science is developed. A guided review and application of research methodologies is a central theme to doctoral education. Students examine a nursing phenomenon with the guidance of nursing theory to apprise clinical decision-making and nursing interventions. A key to the doctoral-prepared nurse's contribution to the profession is the opportunity to generate new nursing theories and test existing theories for practice. A component to this contribution is the doctoral-prepared nurse being skilled in comparing and contrasting various approaches to theory development and use of theory in practice. Doctoral nursing education ensures the student is exposed to theory's role in nursing science and hence aids in socializing the student to the doctoral role. At the doctoral level, theory is an integral element contributing to the growth and adaptation of nursing science.

From diploma to doctoral preparation, nursing theory is foundational to supporting and growing nursing knowledge. Each level of nursing practice has a unique contribution to the profession. Nursing theory is an influential tool and a grounding framework to guide curriculum, drive research, and promote evidence-based practice.

CHAPTER 3

Creating a New Relationship with the APN

Key Terms

APN clinician: A master's-prepared and certified RN specializing as a nurse practitioner, clinical nurse specialist, or nurse midwife.

Nurse generalist: An RN with an Associate's or Bachelor of Science degree with professional licensure and skills to develop care at any point in the health care network.

APRN compact legislation: Adopted August 12, 2020, it allows an advanced-practice RN to hold one multistate license with a privilege to practice in other compact states.

Clinical nurse leader (CNL): A master's-educated nurse prepared for practice across the continuum of care within any health care setting.

Collaboration: An evolving process that calls for active participation from contributing individuals who engage in shared problem solving and decision-making to achieve a common goal (Hamric et al., 2014).

Concept (nursing): A word or phrase that summarizes the essential characteristics of a phenomenon (Fawcett, 2000).

Evidence based practice: The integration of best research evidence, clinical research, and patient values in making decisions about the care of individual patients (AACN, 2011).

Holistic (holism): The practice of "healing the whole person." This means that nurses should consider a patient's body, mind, spirit, culture, socioeconomic background, and environment when delivering care (American Holistic Nurses Association, n.d.).

Lifelong learning: A dynamic process that encompasses both personal and professional life (Davis et al., 2014).

Metacognition: A process in which cognitive patients recognize, monitor, feedback and adjust many cognitive factors that affect their own psychological states, task objectives, and learning strategies (Flavell, 1979).

Nursing phenomena: Nursing theories focus on the phenomena of nursing and nursing care. A phenomenon is the term, description, or label given to describe an idea or responses about an event, a situation, a process, a group of events, or a group of situations (Meleis, 2011). This phenomenon may be temporary or permanent.

Pedagogy: The art and science of teaching, instruction, and training (Horsfall et al., 2012).

Philosophy: An approach to nursing created by an individual nurse in their daily practice based on the nurse's personal beliefs of what nursing is, the role nursing plays in the health care environment, and how the nurse creates a nurse–patient relationship.

Translational research: Research aimed at enhancing the adoption of best practices in the community (AACN, 2011).

Introduction

APNs are vital contributors to health care delivery, leading nursing forward, and ensuring competency of future nurses, which is steadfast in providing quality, safe, and current evidenced-based care. However, present definitions of an APN may limit contributions to the overall profession and the strength of how health care is delivered and how nurses are led and educated. There are numerous roles RNs engage in at the bedside, as many nurses can attest, such as advocate and teacher. A similar alignment can be seen in the roles of the APN. To provide a working definition of an APN, a review of an existing definition is presented.

According to the International Council of Nurses (2020), an APN is commonly used on a global scale for nurse practitioners and clinical nurse specialists who have acquired an expert knowledge base, clinical competencies, and complex decision-making skills at an advanced level. In examination of the International Council of Nurses definition, a prerequisite tends to rest in higher education preparation, with a minimal master's degree in nursing along with a career trajectory that specializes in a specific professional setting. For purposes of this text and to support the academic preparations of students in graduate programs, an APN is an RN enrolled in a Master of Nursing program with a focus on clinical practice, leadership, and education.

The definition of an APN rests in their chief responsibilities, which include preventative care, disease management, education, and leadership while holding key characteristics such as continual learning, proficient communication, and scientific aptitude. Master's-prepared nurses are engaged in clinical practice, leadership, and education acquiring an expert level of working knowledge within their specialties and who are engaged in ongoing critical thinking to enhance their specialty role. For the purpose of this text and to enlighten APNs on the applied use of nursing theory, a practical definition of the APN, theory's unique contributions, APNs commitment to lifelong learning, and ultimately adopting a community of practice will be presented through the roles of clinician, leader, and educator.

The chapter will address the following learning objectives:

1. Describe the health care contributions of the APN through the roles of clinician, leader, and educator.
2. Explore nursing theory's relationship in assisting the APN through the roles of clinician, leader, and educator.
3. Illustrate the APNs commitment to lifelong learning through specific practices to adopt a community of practice.

Clarifying the Role of the APN

APN roles are undeniably essential to quality care and patient outcomes. Advanced nursing practice is based on critical thinking and understanding the required theoretical background (Parker & Hill, 2017). Nursing has its own philosophical and theoretical foundation, which is bolstered by a comprehensive research base comprised of innovative practice frameworks, interventions, and care models (Stucky et al., 2020). Thus, nursing provides great value in the provision of care in collaboration with other disciplines (Stucky et al., 2020). Despite these opportunities for nursing, professional identities and role clarity may elude nursing and create inaccurate perceptions within other interprofessional disciplines. As health care becomes fragmented and increasingly multifaceted, leading health care organizations such as the Institute of Medicine (IOM) have recommended and supported interprofessional collaboration. The process of interprofessional collaboration is not without challenges as it requires a clear delineation of roles and professional boundaries. Health care professionals need to be able to identify and counter discourses and conversations concerning the ANP role so that the role can develop and be used to its full potential to enhance health care provision (Thompson & McNamara, 2021).

APN Clinician

An APN clinician can take on different roles, from the nurse practitioner to the clinical nurse specialist and certified nurse midwife. Most consider the APN to fall into one of these roles; however, the text will set a wider net on the nurse leader and educator as part of an advanced practice nurse role. In the last decade, guidelines have been established and promoted under the consensus model of APRN regulation: licensure, accreditation, certification, and education. The efforts of professional organizations, such as the National Organization of Nurse Practitioner Faculties (NONPF), American Association of Nurse Practitioners (AANP), and the National Association of Clinical Nurse Specialists (NACNS), have made positive strides to present a clear understanding of the roles sought by nurse practitioners and clinical nurse specialists.

The guidelines support a master's or doctoral degree as minimum entry into practice with the addition of credentialing as a function of regulation. These established guidelines assist others, such as policymakers, to better understand the role of the clinical-based APN. The NP and the clinical nurse specialist (CNS) can specialize in their clinical settings, much like a nurse generalist can further expand specialized nursing care. As graduate prepared and certified within their unique specialties, APN clinicians influence not only the nursing profession, but also impact the productivity of working with other health care disciplines and influence public perceptions of health care providers. Their roles are palpable to health care delivery and directly impact health care key indicators and patient outcomes. Even before the COVID-19 pandemic, the NP's position in health care was widespread, with millions of U.S. patients choosing NPs as their health care provider, comprising 1.06 billion patient visits in 2018 (AANP, 2020).

Check Out These Links

- Consensus Model of APRN Regulation: Licensure, Accreditation, Certification, and Education: https://ncsbn.org/papers/consensus-model-for-aprn-regulation-licensure-accreditation-certification-and-education
- National Organization of Nurse Practitioner Faculties: https://www.nonpf.org/
- American Association of Nurse Practitioners: https://www.aanp.org/
- National Association of Clinical Nurse Specialists: https://nacns.org/

The nursing profession strives to create a unique identity and advance its practice into multiple specialty roles. An example of a national misunderstanding of the role of advanced practice clinicians has resulted in the absence of nurse practitioner full practice authority in 28 states. Nurse practitioners are fully prepared to provide needed primary and acute care services while meeting the demands of underrepresented populations. The COVID-19 pandemic unmasked an even greater necessity to clarify APN roles to appreciate each APNs contributions to improving a complex health care system. The pandemic may have pushed for emergency responses but also began a new era for the nurse practitioner by expanding the scope of practice through emergency regulatory policy changes (Stucky et al., 2020). The necessity to do so has created further role confusion but has also stimulated new opportunities for the NP. Despite the temporary policy and regulatory changes, the NP has the prospect to advocate for full practice authority in their state (APRN compact legislation) by increasing public and political awareness of NPs value in optimal patient health outcomes. Beyond the advanced practice clinician's direct patient care role, the effect of full-practice authority for the NP is supported by the long history of nursing's collective body of knowledge from academia to clinical practice while offering unique insights to shape health care policy.

APRN Compact Legislation

For more information on APRN Compact Legislation, please visit the following links:

- https://www.ncsbn.org/compacts/aprn-compact.page
- https://www.aanp.org/advocacy/advocacy-resource/position statements/aprn-compact-licensure
- https://www.aprncompact.com/

APN Leader

Leaders are found in every area of the workplace, and nursing is no exception. All clinical and nonclinical settings that involve nursing have leaders to guide and inspire work toward a common goal(s). According to Catton (2020), the health care environment can be characterized by increasing costs, budget cuts, staffing shortages, an aging population, high-demand work environment, increasing patient acuity, and the emergence of new diseases, hence making the role of the nurse leader one of the most vital positions in health care. There is a demand for nurse leaders to embrace innovation and creative thinking to respond to the multiple challenges faced daily. There has never been more demand for nurse leadership than during the COVID-19 pandemic. The quick actions of nurses to respond in crisis mode placed leadership and communication skills at the forefront of nursing practice. Nurse leaders were required to use enhanced skill sets to prioritize and promote cognitive, behavioral, and emotional responses among staff (Fowler & Robbins, 2022). The nurse leader has the potential to impact health care practices in a way that upholds the moral and ethical tenets of the nursing profession. The need for strong nurse leaders will remain steadfast, requiring nurses to consider positions of leadership to engage in ongoing professional development, interprofessional education, collaboration, and outcome-based practice to meet the needs of today's patient.

To further demonstrate the necessity for nurse leaders, the IOM's report, *The Future of Nursing: Leading Change, Advancing Health*, supports education programs for leadership development to prepare nurses at all levels to be part of the decision-making process to transform the health care system. As part of the IOM's recommendations, a call is made for nurses, nursing educational programs, and nursing associations to prepare the nursing workforce to assume leadership positions across all levels. The IOM has set a precedent for health care systems to ensure nurses are provided the opportunities to work within leadership roles.

Knowing the need for nurse leadership is one part of the equation; however, defining nurse leadership can be seen though identification of characteristics and skills required of nurse leaders. Hughes (2018) reviewed 10 national and international research studies to identify the characteristics of great nurse leaders. The leadership characteristics identified were integrity, accessibility, motivation of others, emotional capability, and social intelligence. Skills needed to achieve these characteristics include a commitment to excellence, passion for their work, clear vision, strategic focus, trustworthiness, respectfulness, approachability, empathy, caring, and commitment to coaching and development of staff (Brunt & Bogdan, 2023). In consensus, leaders serve as role models and motivate others through empowerment, accessibility to resources, and recognition of contributions.

Multiple avenues exist for the nurse to enter leadership. These include nursing leadership in clinical settings, administrative and managerial leadership, and advanced practice. The AACN (2013) has outlined the need for clinical nurse leaders to take on the role of change agents and innovators. Beyond the supervision of staff, nurse leaders have responsibilities in addressing ethical standards, organizational analysis, economic viability, strategic governance, and change management—all of which are critical to making positive changes required to ensure patient safety, quality care, and effective interprofessional collaboration.

APN Leadership Organizations

Check out the following links:

- American Organization for Nursing Leadership (AONL): https://www.aonl.org/resources/nurse-leader-competencies
- The Association for Nursing Professional Development: https://www.anpd.org/

APN Educator

The nurse educator is an advocate for the nurse by promoting nursing practice through the application of scientific inquiries, EBP, and research into nursing curriculum to prepare students to navigate and practice within the profession. Nurse educators hold advanced degrees, either a master's or doctoral degree. The role of the nurse educator is pivotal in preparing nurses at all levels to practice with current knowledge, critical thinking. judgment, and skills to safely apply nursing practice within a selected clinical specialty.

The World Health Organization (WHO, 2023) outlines eight competencies for nurse educators: theories and principles of adult learning, curriculum design and implementation, nursing practice, research and evidence, communication, collaboration, ethical and legal principles of the profession, monitoring, evaluation, management, leadership, and advocacy. The competencies laid forth by the WHO complement many of the same characteristics and skills described for the APN in clinician and leadership positions. The National League for Nursing (NLN) issued the need for nurse educators, which is equivalent to the need for nurses now and in the future. The U.S. Bureau of Labor Statistics (2022) projects the U.S. health care systems will have almost 200,000 openings for nurses though the year 2030. In addition to the rising need for nurses, the National Advisory Council on Nurse Education and Practice cited a 7.2% vacancy rate for full-time nursing faculty, which also resulted in nursing schools turning aways more than 80,000 qualified student applicants in 2019 (National Advisory Council on Nurse Education and Practice [NACNEP], 2021). Like other industries, proficient education of nursing professionals is essential to the future of health care. According to the American Association of Colleges of Nursing (AACN, n.d.), education has a significant impact on the knowledge and competencies of nurses and other healthcare providers.

According to the NLN (2022), nurse educators are in a unique position to make an impact by inspiring nurses in training and by promoting public health through work in schools, businesses, hospitals, and community agencies. Nurse educators are skilled in intellectual stimulation by knowing the latest research. Nurse educators are key to incorporating research trends and findings to inspire students toward innovative thinking as part of the skill set needed to enter today's health care environment.

APN Educator Organizations

Check out the following website links:

- NLN: https://www.yearofnurseeducators.org/
- AACN: https://www.aacnnursing.org/

Theory: Assisting the APN's Role as Clinician, Leader, and Educator

Nurses often wander how theory plays a role in their nursing profession. From frontline care providers whose interactions with patients creates opportunities to improve health care delivery to the leader who steers policy and creates a work culture of teamwork, and finally to the educator who teaches and models those with vested interest in becoming nurses and APNs, theory is an essential tool. Nursing has a pulse on the patient experience, its professional trajectory, and the education needs of future care providers. Nurses who embrace nursing theory can implement care interventions, professional standards, and quality curriculum that appreciates the needs of the patient, the health care organization, and the student.

Theory plays an integral role in nursing actions regardless of clinical specialties by speaking to a broad range of nursing phenomena. In order to understand nursing phenomena, it is important to gain insight on a concept (of nursing). A concept is a word or phrase that summarizes the essential characteristics of a phenomenon (Fawcett, 2000). A phenomenon is the term, description, or label given to describe an idea or responses about an event, a situation, a process, a group of events, or a group of situations (Meleis, 2011). APNs who are aware of nursing phenomena can align theory to guide their practice in each APN role: clinician, leader, and educator.

Examples of Nursing Phenomena

- Self-care in nursing
- Compassion fatigue
- Moral distress
- Nurse advocacy

- End of life
- Quality of life
- Nurse burnout
- Situational awareness
- Competence
- Empowerment
- Comfort
- Resilience

APN's expanded responsibilities and scopes of practice place them in a heightened position to utilize theory and open dialogue for theory's application in today's health care and social, political, and academic environments. In the APN's unique contributions to people's health and to inspire those who care for others, nursing theory impacts the APN's ability to describe, assess, and plan for patient treatment through a holistic lens. In close examination of the APN roles of clinician, leader, and educator, we can see the role theory has in assisting the APN in developing specialized knowledge to further enhance the APN in professional practice.

APN Clinician

As APN clinicians hold expanded authority and scope of practice, theory becomes predominant in decision-making. At the core of the APN clinician's practice is how knowledge is used. Nursing practice is described as goal-directed, deliberative, action-oriented, and coordinated work for and with people to enhance healthful living or peaceful dying (Kim, 2010). Clinical judgment and decision-making are critical responsibilities for the APN clinician and impact patient care experiences and outcomes. Theory provides a guide for APN clinicians to assist in the decision-making process. An APN clinician can apply theory through a developed nursing practice philosophy and through specific clinical situations.

Theory reminds the APN clinician of maintaining a nursing focus while assuring a commitment to a nursing philosophy in practice. Theory offers the APN a focused direction for clinical practice by orienting to fundamental nursing philosophies and attributes. The APN formulates a nursing practice philosophy to influence actions, reactions, and reflections of their clinical practice. A philosophy is formed out of the APN's education, practice history (or Carper's personal knowing) and beliefs and values regarding patient care ethics; hence, nursing theory and philosophies are directly related and affect one another. An APN clinician's philosophy will be attracted to related theories and models based on clinical specialties and personal values.

Student Activity: Identifying Personal Nursing Philosophy

A nursing philosophy captures your beliefs and goals as a practicing nurse and future APN. Philosophies are fluid as you engage in different specialties and advance your education. Creating a nursing philosophy and adjusting your philosophy as you advance your career is a positive way to reflect ethical care, beliefs, and theories, which are the basis your clinical nursing practice.

Reflect

Review concepts, theories, and models of nursing and use reflection to consider personal ways of knowing in nursing along with past and current nursing practice experiences to determine a philosophy of nursing practice for your future role as an APN. Recognize personal values and beliefs you hold within your nursing practice(s).

Summarize

Using a journal, write down significant experiences you have had in your field of nursing. Recognize your strengths and weaknesses. Identify specific concepts in these experiences. Align those concepts with nursing theories.

Create

Use the template to write a brief and succinct personal nursing philosophy statement:

- Serving as a _________ nurse means _________ and by using my knowledge in _________, I want to _________.

In addition to developing a nursing practice philosophy, APNs should reflect on the purpose of theory. APNs can selectively use nursing theories to assist in explaining and understanding clinical situations.

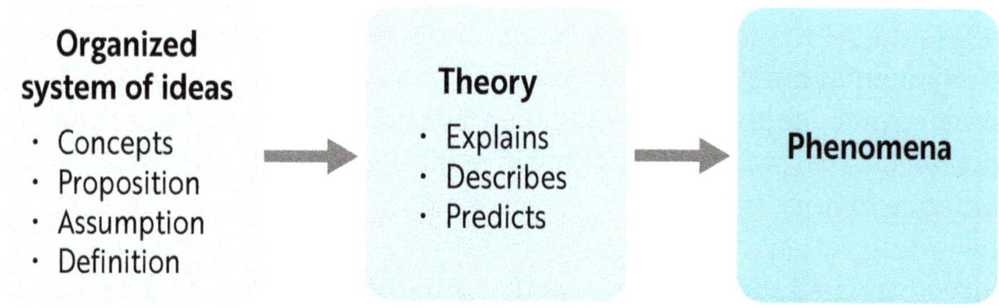

FIGURE 3.1 What is nursing theory?

Clinical situations are unique from each other as much as the patient experience is unique. The use of theory for the APN clinician becomes selective to the clinical situation by guiding the APN to explain and understand what is working and what is not working. It is important to note no one theory can fit all situations and it takes knowledge of many nursing theories and models to address different clinical situations. Selected theories and the APN clinician's knowledge work in concert with one another to carry out deliberate action and decision-making to address patient needs.

TABLE 3.1 Example: Nurse Practitioner Nursing Practice Philosophy and Selection of Theory to Guide Care

NP Philosophy	Specific Clinical Situation	Theory-Guided Practice	Rationale for Use of Theory
Tim, CRNP-BC, has adopted a personal nursing practice philosophy that assumes NPs promote health from a holistic viewpoint with or without the absence of disease.	Joe, the patient, is struggling to quit smoking after 25 years. Joe is recently divorced and lives in an apartment building on the fifth floor with limited use of a working elevator.	Pender's health promotion model that assumes health is a positive dynamic state and self-initiated change of individual and environmental characteristics is essential to changing behavior.	Using a holistic approach to care, Tim will assess Joe's biopsychosocial influences in assisting and those influences that create challenges to quitting smoking. Tim, NP, will guide Joe to understand effects of smoking on health and how to employ actions to quit smoking and add exercise to promote health, such as using stairs in his apartment building.

In addition, it is important to mention how health care systems have employed nursing theories to organizational mission and philosophies. Health care systems who have earned a Magnet designation strive to integrate nursing theories into policies and procedures to ensure best practices are utilized and evaluated. The designation of Magnet hospital is awarded by the American Nurses Credentialing Center (ANCC) for health care systems who have met goals in excellence and professionalism. A major attraction for health care systems to earn a Magnet designation is to provide excellent nursing care with a higher retention of nursing staff. Nurses employed in Magnet health care systems are skilled in disseminating best practices in nursing care. Best practices are accomplished through research's foundation or alignment to nursing theory by recognizing a nursing phenomenon and seeking best practice to address these issues through nursing care practices.

Magnet Recognition

- A pathway to nursing excellence/care that utilizes nursing strategic goals to improve an organization's patient outcomes.
  - https://www.nursingworld.org/organizational-programs/magnet/

APN Leader

Nursing has the opportunity to inspire leadership in many areas of clinical or educational practices. Leadership is a complex and multifaceted role, and many nurses pursue graduate degrees to assist in identifying and navigating leadership roles within the nursing profession. Nursing leadership has evolved by distinguishing from previous perceptions of management to directing actions toward positive impacts on health care delivery based on evidence. An opportunity exists for the APN leader to foster nurses to influence health care through innovation and science-based practice. APN leaders can use both leadership theories, such as the transformational leadership theory by James MacGregor Burns, and nursing theories to guide their responsibilities from fiscal management to creating synergy in the workplace to meet organizational (shared) goals. A review of leadership theories and styles with an alignment to some nursing theories is provided as an example of the relationship between both.

As health care systems encounter daily challenges, it is important for nurse leaders to be aware of the changing workforce. Multiple generations work in the nursing profession, which can create opportunities for nurse leaders to motivate diverse thinking and collaboration to insert highly effective and efficient teams. Studies have demonstrated there is a correlation between nurses' perceptions of their administration's competency to their own job satisfaction (Ulrich et al., 2019). With the impact from the COVID-19 pandemic, nurse leaders are in demand to be accountable for budgets and patient satisfaction and for ensuring nursing staff are equipped, both in skill competency and with equipment, to meet the demands of the health care environment. Concepts such as mentoring, coaching, being authentic, resilience, and empowerment have become central to the education and ongoing competencies for the APN leader.

TABLE 3.2 APN Leader: Aligning Leadership Style and Theories to Nursing Theories

Leadership Style/Theory	Assumption(s)	Alignment to Nursing Theory
Transformational leadership	A relationship between the leader and the follower exists to motivate each other to higher levels, resulting in value system congruence between the leader and the follower (Krishnn, 2002).	*Peplau's theory of interpersonal relations*: Four phases of the nurse–patient (staff) relationship can be utilized to engage in information seeking (orientation phase), build trust (identification phase), problem solve (exploitation phase), and support independence in practice (resolution phase). Peplau's theory can be used by nurse leaders to engage staff in the change process.
Transactional leadership	Transactional leadership is task focused and involves short-term goals, is focused on contingent reward, and involves management by exception, whereby the leader intervenes only when necessary (Richards, 2020).	*Orlando's deliberative nursing process theory*: The nurse–patient situation is dynamic; actions and reactions are influenced by both the nurse and the patient. The model revolves around five major interrelated concepts: the function of professional nursing, presenting behavior, immediate reaction, nursing process discipline, and improvement.
Authentic leadership	A style that focuses on how leaders can use relationships to enable people to find meaning at work, developing trust and optimism, promoting inclusive and healthy work environments, and encouraging honest relationships (Richards, 2020).	*Boykin and Schoenhofer's theory of nursing as caring: A model for transforming practice*: As an expression of nursing, caring is the intentional and authentic presence of the nurse with another person who is recognized as living caring and growing in caring. Nursing is a shared relationship.
Ethical leadership	A style in which leaders act with respect for values and beliefs and demonstrate honesty, fairness, and integrity (Richards, 2020).	*Leininger's transcultural nursing theory*: Values, beliefs, and practices for culturally related care are shaped by, and often embedded in, "the worldview, language, religious (or spiritual), kinship (social), political (or legal), educational, economic, technological, ethnohistorical, and environmental context of the culture" (Leininger, 2002, p. 190).

(Continued)

TABLE 3.2 APN Leader: Aligning Leadership Style and Theories to Nursing Theories (*Continued*)

Leadership Style/Theory	Assumption(s)	Alignment to Nursing Theory
Collective leadership	A style in which formal and informal leaders work together to generate actions (Richards, 2020).	*Travelbee's human-to-human relationship model*: The purpose of nursing is to help and support an individual, family, or community to prevent or cope with the struggles of illness and suffering and, if necessary, to find significance in these occurrences, with the ultimate goal being the presence of hope.

APN Educator

APN educators inspire, teach, and mentor the next generation of nurses and APNs. Staying current in EBP, research, and health care trends, APN educators play a fundamental position in equipping tomorrow's care providers. APN educators are vital in both academic and clinical settings and are responsible for being experts to build partnerships with health care settings to ensure students receive adequate care experiences. Educators foster growth for both the student and the health care setting by being servant leaders, patient advocates, and research partners.

Nursing has accepted theory as basic to its practice, and thus theory becomes a critical component to curriculum development. Theory can serve as a framework for curriculum development and be taught as foundations of concepts throughout a program's curriculum. As health care landscapes change at rapid paces and with influences from nursing regulatory standards, health care economic challenges, and stakeholder demands, concepts of nursing and competency-based curriculum are navigating curriculum development. The AACN (n.d.a.) has re-envisioned essentials, or standards, for professional nursing education. In this re-envisioning of educational standards, 10 domains with hundreds of sub-competencies have been established to guide nursing programs at all levels of nursing preparation. Concepts of nursing practice were identified as transferrable knowledge to enhance learning, allowing students to make connections to nursing practice. Some of the concepts identified include clinical judgment, SDOH, communication, and ethics. With the inclusion of a competency-based approach to nursing education, students are provided with the prerequisites to practice and meet the health care system's expectations of graduates.

AACN Essentials

For more information on the AACN Essentials, please check out the link:

- https://dev.aacnnursing.org/Essentials

With the expectations from health care and nursing organizational standards, APN educators are indispensable in preparing nurses to meet daily challenges with exceptional clinical judgment and care interventions to promote the best possible health outcomes for patients. Nurse educators utilize theory in multiple teaching dimensions. Some nursing theories, such as Faye Abdellah's 21 nursing problems and Virginia Henderson's need theory, were developed to guide nursing curriculums so that students could implement a systematic method to assess and address patient needs while implementing care interventions under the framework of nursing.

TABLE 3.3 APN Clinician, Leader, and Educator Curriculum Mapping to Nursing Theory

Nursing Theory	Purpose	Implementation: APN Clinician (AC) APN Leader (AL) APN Educator (AE)
Virginia Henderson's Need Theory	To teach nurses to develop effective and therapeutic care plans to promote patient's recovery	AC engages the patient to independence by addressing a holistic assessment of the patient's needs AL creates and maintains a work environment that supports nurses' work and ensures resources needed for specific patient population needs AE establishes a teaching plan to incorporate theoretical assumptions to assess and assist students in creating an appropriate patient care plan
Faye Abdellah's 21 Nursing Problems	To assist with the diagnosis process through nursing's assessments and caring interventions by being focused on the 21 nursing problems to develop plans of care that address the developmental, emotional, and physical needs of the patient	AC accurately and systematically assesses patient needs to apply appropriate treatments to address illness/health diagnoses AL creates and maintains a work environment that focuses on patient-centered care AE implements teaching plans to engage students in intellectual competencies and technical skills to care for patients across the life span

(Continued)

TABLE 3.3 APN Clinician, Leader, and Educator Curriculum Mapping to Nursing Theory (*Continued*)

Nursing Theory	Purpose	Implementation: APN Clinician (AC) APN Leader (AL) APN Educator (AE)
Dorothea Orem's Theory of Nursing Systems	To facilitate a patient's level of self-care to effectively perform activities to maintain personal health and well-being	AC assesses, educates, and supports patients to understand their illness and move forward with maintenance of disease to a level of self-care that promotes a sense of health and well-being AL guides staff and interdisciplinary partners to engage in comprehensive patient care that promotes self-efficacy and improved patient outcomes AE instructs students on how to promote a patient's personal development and when to take action to care for the patient while demonstrating support on how to cope with obstacles in their path to health and wellness
Madeleine Leininger's Culture Care Theory	To affirm and address a patient's needs based on culture and care toward health and wellness	AC is aware and actively engaged in understanding cultures and associated values and beliefs to provide culture-specific care AL role models and provides learning opportunities for staff to continue growth in culturally competent care AE provides students with clinical settings that offer opportunities to care for patients of many cultures and assesses understanding of culturally competent care by integrating cultures in various learning strategies

TABLE 3.3 APN Clinician, Leader, and Educator Curriculum Mapping to Nursing Theory (*Continued*)

Nursing Theory	Purpose	Implementation: APN Clinician (AC) APN Leader (AL) APN Educator (AE)
Hildegard Peplau's Interpersonal Relations Theory	To engage in building a therapeutic nurse–patient relationship through mutual respect and trust	AC engages in a therapeutic relationship with the patient through skilled interview and communication skills AL utilizes interpersonal skills with staff, patients, and interdisciplinary colleagues to assess for needs within the work environment AE incorporates the theory's phases of interpersonal relations, orientation, identification, exploitation, and resolution, to guide students through the process of developing an effective relationship with the patient to best meet their immediate needs

Nursing theory can be used in more ways than curriculum development and creation of learning strategies. Nursing theory can guide the APN educator to develop a personal philosophy of educating others in the practice of nursing. Theory guides educators on how to reach students at their unique level of understanding and learning style. Much like the concept of patient-centered care, educators focus teaching efforts on how to reach students and engage them in the learning process which best suits their learning needs. As nurse educators engage in various pedagogies, the educator must also be aware of the changing demographics and generational thinking among students entering the nursing profession. Just as patient demographics change, so does the student body, resulting in educators needing to stay innovative in teaching practices to ensure students are provided a sound educational experience to learn and flourish.

Making the Commitment to Lifelong Learning

Nurses will periodically evaluate their career path and often decide on a new trajectory, which may require learning new skills, completing a certification, or advancing academic preparations. It may go without saying, nurses by nature are lifelong learners. Even amid landmark reports, such as the IOM's, *The Future of Nursing: Leading Change, Advancing Health*, nursing has strongly encouraged its practitioners to advance their education as indicated by BSN-prepared nurses being studied and resulting in improved patient outcomes (Aiken, 2014). What exactly is lifelong learning and, principally, what does it mean to the advanced practice nurse?

"Lifelong learning in nursing is defined as a dynamic process, which encompasses both personal and professional life" (Davis et al., 2014, p. 441). As this definition opens the dialogue for everyone, nursing may view the concept differently based on each nurse's practice environment and unique knowledge gained through personal knowing. Nurses who decide to change career trajectories will seek new knowledge and perspectives affiliated with their selected environment. This is when the APN plays a key role in nurturing their individual and colleague learning as a continuous process.

The concept of lifelong learning should be clarified. To fully encompass the qualities of lifelong learning, it is important to distinguish the process as active and ongoing. Once nurses can value the active process, characteristics of lifelong learners can be recognized. These include reflection (metacognition), questioning, enjoyment of learning, understanding the dynamic nature of knowledge, and seeking learning opportunities (Davis et al., 2014). As APNs seek advanced academic preparation in the areas of clinician, leader, and educator, methodologies to inspire ongoing pursuits of knowledge will be presented. A three-prong approach is introduced for the APN to engage in continuous learning in both their specialized fields as well as in the dynamic culture of the health care environment. The approach will consist of the following prescriptions:

- Becoming an avid reader of current discipline and health care literature
- Creating a thinking diary
- Adopting a community of practice by employing actions of thinking out loud and open dialogue with colleagues and other interdisciplinary healthcare professionals

Becoming an Avid Reader of Current Discipline and Health Care Literature

Nursing and medical literature are at the heart of expanding knowledge to enhance individual practice and safeguard quality patient care. As research is significant in directing nursing practice, becoming an avid reader is a necessary responsibility and skill for the APN. Nursing literature aims to answer focused questions, inform clinicians, influence policies, and identify future research endeavors. Each area speaks directly to the APN clinician, leader, and educator.

Translational research and EBP are the professional standards for the nurse and the APN. It is imperative for the nurse and nursing student to utilize best practices to drive nursing actions. In 2013, the information literacy competency standards for nursing were established to address the information skills necessary for nursing students at associate's, baccalaureate, master's, and doctoral levels and are written for nursing faculty and librarians who support nursing programs and nursing students in academic settings (Association of College & Research Libraries, 2018). The purpose of the standards is to provide a framework for faculty and students to support information literacy skills and promote lifelong learning. Five standards are presented to guide the student and faculty to adopt value in the need for continuous improvements based on new knowledge (Association of College & Research Libraries, 2018).

Information Literacy Competency Standards for Nursing

For more information on the five standards for students and faculty to gain on information literacy skills, please see provided link:

- https://www.ala.org/acrl/standards/nursing

The most effective way to gain new knowledge for the APN is to become research literate. Reading research to gain insight into the trending investigations can invigorate the APN in practice. For the clinician, it can lead to implementation of new standardized practice protocols; for the leader, it can stimulate dialogue among interdisciplinary colleagues on policy development; and for the educator, it drives curriculum changes and responses to student inquisitions of best practices. Nursing literature is an excellent means to learn about the discipline of nursing in context to health care challenges. Through avid reading, the APN can appreciate the movement of the discipline to differentiating itself and ensuring a holistic perspective remains at the forefront of research and practice.

To begin the process of becoming an avid reader of nursing literature, it is important to understand and employ skills in literature reviews. A literature review is also known as a retrospective survey. There are multiple approaches to a literature review:

- *Narrative review*: Based on an author's (expert) subjective review, addressing a specific question with a summary of findings. This type of review may lead to biased summaries; however, these may demonstrate avenues for further literature based on a specific topic of research.

- *Integrative review*: Utilizes data from experimental and nonexperimental research studies to define concepts, review theories, and analyze methodologies.
- *Systematic review*: A comprehensive and extensive process to identify and summarize a focused clinical question.
- *Meta-analysis*: A statistical approach combining data from a systematic review. The main purpose is to increase the data quantitatively, and hence statistical power, to determine results of a treatment or intervention.

Each type of literature review can assist the APN in exploring new ideas, research questions, and potentially best practices to employ in their area of specialty. Beginning the process should start with conducting a literature review to identify relevant topics, issues, and/or concerns within selected areas of nursing practice. Using a simple four-step approach can aid the APN in locating relevant and current literature.

TABLE 3.4 Applying Steps of a Literature Review

1. Organizing topic(s) into concepts.	**2. Identify databases.**	**3. Develop search terms.**	**4. Practice search skills.**
Write down clinical issues or concerns and relate nursing concepts to the topics to help formulate inclusion and exclusion criteria for a literature search.	Consider databases to search for topics that may yield the most results.	Create a PICO (person, problem, intervention, comparison, and outcome) framework to assist in narrowing search terms.	Utilize Boolean operators AND/OR to develop a search.

Creating a Thinking Diary

As APNs begin to read literature as part of their commitment to lifelong learning, oftentimes topics, new knowledge, or ideas for future research may become scattered. Creating a personal thinking diary can aid the APN in tracking ideas and knowledge, especially during times of transition. Free-flowing and nonjudgmental thinking can be a liberating experience for the nurse and the APN. By collecting critical thinking in the modality of notes, the nurse and APN can be free to explore ideas and suggestions for practice and possible future research endeavors. Part of this tracking process can be a means to organizing found resources related to a topic of interest.

An area of further exploration in this book will include the concept of metacognition. A thinking diary can be a place where metacognition can live and provide direction for applying new knowledge and brainstorming innovative solutions. Oftentimes the nurse or APN experiences are confusing and intimidating. Having a process and a place to make sense of these experiences affords the nurse an opportunity to grow and learn. In the thinking diary, the APN can navigate current practices, research trends, and their own values or biases in any given situation. This valuable time of reflection is another way for APNs to provide themselves with self-care.

APN Thinking Diary Content Suggestions

- List APA references of literature read.
- Include themes, concepts, and topics associated with each article.
- Map the literature to your own ideas and topics of concern.
- Provide a space of introspection on the article's contents as it relates to your own nursing experiences.
- Explore Carper's patterns of knowing specific to your current nursing practice.
- Provide space to describe your feelings, biases, and connection (or not) to personal beliefs you experienced with a specific situation.
- Summarize your (ongoing) achievements and goals (met or unmet).
- Provide a space to explore your strengths, weaknesses, opportunities, and threats.
- Provide a space for innovative thinking to discover possible solutions and future research ideas.

Adopting a Community of Practice

Adopting a community practice is a concept that promotes discipline and interdisciplinary collaboration. The health care environment is primed for interconnections between health care providers as a result of the COVID-19 pandemic. The impact of the pandemic shifted health care to a team approach out of necessity; however, the effects of this collaboration can be positive and spearhead interprofessional collaboration on a new level of effective, efficient, and patient-centered teamwork. Nursing has been a champion of interprofessional collaboration and once again can be a leader in this effort to showcase the sharing of information and ideas to better support the patient.

The evidence for collaboration exists, with nurses facing the challenges of acute patient assignments, budgetary constraints, and short staffing, to name a few. A refined view of adopting a community of practice can also be a solution and a supportive system for the APN. In this conception of a community of practice, the APN can actively apply a thinking-out-loud and an open-dialogue approach with other disciplinary and interdisciplinary partners.

In thinking out loud, the APN is encouraged to utilize thoughts, ideas, perceptions identified from the thinking diary to better enhance individual understanding of concepts they wish to explore. For example, an APN clinician may want to explore financial viability for an independent practice as compared to time spent per patient. The APN leader may want to explore caseload and quality of care for underrepresented groups. The APN educator may want to explore learning strategies to teach clinical judgment. All topics were influenced by professional experiences and through avid reading of current nursing literature. Each APN is encouraged to think out loud with other stakeholders in their specialty. The APN clinician can discuss the idea with other primary care providers in independent practice, the APN leader can discuss the idea with other health care system administrators, and the APN educator can discuss the idea with dedicated educational units or clinical sites. In this process of thinking out loud, the APN builds a web of connections and respected input.

To complete this adoption of a community of practice, the APN can engage colleagues in open dialogue to gain perceptions and ideas and to further understand current standards of practice to better enhance their own assessment of their selected topic/issue or concern. Not only can interdisciplinary dialogue create quality patient care, it can also have positive impacts on workplace culture and individual career satisfaction. Setting a wider net on one's learning opportunities can be rewarding for both parties and creates a sense of partnership. The sharing of knowledge and ideas is one definite way to make a commitment to lifelong learning.

Figure Credit

Fig. 3.1: Maye Serrano, "Diagram about Theory," https://rnspeak.com/what-is-a-nursing-theory/. Copyright © 2018 by RNSpeak.com.

PART II

Preparing the APN for Theory-Guided Practice

The APN clinician, leader, and educator's preparation to serve as repositories of nursing knowledge and mentors of evidence-based practice must be grounded in nursing theory. Preparing APNs to use their role, scope of practice, and critical thinking will require new ideas to integrate evidence into practice. Theory is a tool to support APNs to generate innovative concepts to address formidable challenges, whether in clinical care, leading nurses and staff, or in educating future generations of nurses. In addition to being educated to practice in autonomous roles, the APN maintains holistic caring practice as extensions of nursing and not medicine. The APN student will learn the medical model, assume a transformational leadership role, and embrace pedagogical methods of teaching. As the APN student engages in this transformation of advanced skills and knowledge, the commitment to helping others prevent disease, promote health, and connect communities remains bound to the core theoretical underpinnings of the nursing profession.

CHAPTER 4

Pausing to Appreciate the Pandemic's Impact

Key Terms

Artificial intelligence (AI): "A wide-ranging branch of computer science concerned with building smart machines capable of performing tasks that typically require human intelligence" (Christopher, 2020, para 1).

Change agents: People who introduce innovations into a client system that they expect will have consequences that will be desirable, direct, and anticipated Interprofessional Education(E. M. Rogers et al., 2003).

Digital divide: A phenomenon that refers to disparities in information and communications technology access, usage, and outcomes (Lythreatis et al., 2021).

Health disparities: Preventable differences in health outcomes and the opportunity to achieve optimal health (U.S. Government Accountability Office, 2021).

Interdisciplinary care: Team members from different disciplines working collaboratively, with a common purpose, to set goals, make decisions and share resources and responsibilities (Nancarrow et al., 2013).

Predictive analytics: Use of AI to develop predictive algorithms that make individualized diagnostic or prognostic risk predictions (Van Calster et al., 2019).

Patient portal: An online tool designed to help patients keep track of health care provider visits, test results, billing, and prescriptions (MedlinePlus Medical Encyclopedia, n.d.).

Sustainable Development Goals (SDGs): Adopted by all United Nations (n.d.) member states in 2015, provide a shared blueprint for peace and prosperity for people and the planet, now and into the future. At its heart are the 17

SDGs, which are an urgent call for action by all countries—developed and developing—in a global partnership.

Team-based care: The ability to apply relationship-building values and the principles of team dynamics to perform effectively in different team roles to plan, deliver, and evaluate patient/population care and population health programs and policies that are safe, timely, efficient, effective, and equitable (Interprofessional Education Collaborative, 2016).

Telemedicine: A platform for the health care provider to care for patients without an in-person office visit. Sometimes referred to as telehealth. telemedicine is done primarily online with internet access on your computer, tablet, or smartphone (Telehealth.HHS.gov, n.d.)

Value-based care (VBC): A health care delivery model in which providers, including hospitals and physicians are paid based on patient health outcomes (Catalyst, 2017).

Value stream: A long-lived series of steps used to create value (Scaled Agile Framework, 2020).

Introduction

In reflection of 2018 and 2019, health care prioritized its flexibility to meet challenges to ease transitions into the next decade. Health care reform was palpable and alive in the mind of administrators, health care providers, and consumers. Policy was structuring to strengthen compliance and advocacy efforts to expand cost considerations along with federal and state policy decisions impacting healthcare delivery. Additionally, health care was expanding in technological advances with artificial intelligence (AI) on the horizon to impact predictive analytics and realizing peak performance standards and goals.

Then, 2020 came. By March of 2020, the world was halted by a virus. COVID-19 invaded the fabric of the nation and drastically altered health care in a way that defined necessity and created confusion and fear. APNs were standing at the precipice of change. Each APN had to move fluidly through pandemic challenges to ensure nursing maintained its integral place in health care while attempting to holistically care, lead, and educate with unwavering fortitude. The role of the APN changed, as did many other health care roles as a result of the pandemic's shock on "the standard approach" to care delivery. To create innovation and opportunities for positive change, it becomes necessary for nursing to reflect on the time before, during, and after the pandemic. This chapter will reflect on APN pre-pandemic roles and highlight changes to APN roles post-pandemic. Five major post-pandemic impacts of health care delivery, remote care, health care costs, poor patient outcomes, health care disparities, and ethical challenges will be discussed in relationship to invigorating APN roles in clinical care, leading change, and educating future care providers.

The chapter will address the following learning objectives:

1. Reflect on pre-pandemic challenges in health care delivery through the lens of APN clinician, leader, and educator roles.
2. Appraise the APN's role transition with respect to five major post-pandemic impacts on health care: health care delivery, remote care, health care costs, poor patient outcomes, health care disparities, and ethical challenges.
3. Conjecture post-pandemic opportunities for health care delivery innovation within the APN clinician, leader, and educator roles.

Health Care's Pre-Pandemic Challenges

In the years prior to the change in decade, health care reform was a persistent topic of concern for politicians, health care systems, providers, and patients alike. Even with the passage of the Affordable Care Act in 2010, health care costs remained high and out of reach for many, but stakeholders took a safeguarding approach. Researchers, investors, insurance companies, administrators, health care providers, and information technologists, to name a few, had a stake in how health care was delivered, ultimately impacting the health care consumer. A definitive health care key performance indicator is patient outcomes. Patient outcomes have been affected from adverse effects of high cost and limited accessibility of care.

An example demonstrating the drive for health care change in the 21st century can be seen in the use of patient data. Health care, pre-pandemic, was focused on improving patient outcomes by integrating big data to drive policy to the point of care. Electronic health records (EHR) had amplified attention to intensify security on patient data while augmenting patients to take active roles in their health maintenance. A study conducted by Han et al. (2019), concluded patient portal interventions were somewhat effective in improving a few psychological outcomes, such as medication adherence and preventative service use; however, there was insufficient evidence to support the use of patient portals to improve clinical outcomes.

Prior to the pandemic, data-driven strategies were at the heart of health care reform. Examples of data-driven health care methods were found in electronic health records, medical imaging, genomic sequencing, payor records, medical and pharmaceutical research, wearable technology, and medical devices. Despite the promises of these strategies, challenges persisted, which included efficient and cost-appropriate software and health information privacy. Since the pandemic, many of the same technology-based strategies have been catapulted to a rapid and robust adoption in health care services.

Applications of Data-Driven Strategies in Health Care Delivery

- Data mining and analytics to identify causes of disease(s)
- Predictive analytics of genetics, lifestyle, and social influences to prevent disease
- Aggregating data to drive personalized care
- Data-driven research in medicine, nursing, and pharmacology to impact patient diagnostics, treatments, and care interventions
- Data to identify medication errors and potential adverse reactions
- Value-based strategies to impact better patient health outcomes
- Big data monitoring to identify disease trends and implement health strategies to respond to changes in demographics, geography, and socioeconomics to impact better community health

The impetus for the use of data-driven approaches is to continue to strive to provide value-based care (VBC). Under a VBC framework, health care providers are rewarded for helping patients improve their health, reduce the effects and incidence of chronic disease, and live healthier lives in an evidence-based way (Catalyst, 2017). Gaining insight into VBC can guide the APN to recognize the relationship VBC has with clinical practice, leadership and management decision-making, and nursing education.

Distinguishing the Difference of Value-Based Care for APNs

- Measuring patient health outcomes against the cost of delivering the outcomes (Catalyst, 2017)
- Lower costs and proven better outcomes
- Higher patient satisfaction
- Stronger cost controls
- Reduced health care spending

Examples of Value-Based Care Models

- **Medical homes**: A coordinated approach to patient care led by a primary care provider who directs patient care with a clinical care team.
- **Accountable care organizations (ACOs)**: Health care providers and hospitals work as a team within a network to deliver the best and most efficient care at the lowest cost possible.
- **Hospital value-based purchasing program (VBP)**: Acute care facilities receive adjusted payments based on the quality of care they deliver.

APNs' Role Pre-Pandemic

As we reflect on the challenges pre-pandemic, it is important to recognize the increasing nursing shortage and the sense of burnout among health care providers. Prominent illustrations can be found in both clinical and nonclinical circumstances. Clinically, health care providers cared for an alarming rise in chronic diseases requiring a multiple disciplinary step approach to health (disease) management. Nonclinically, SDOH impacted people's abilities to live a healthy life. APNs needed to consider a person's literacy level, transportation access, housing, and food security, to name a few. Prior to the pandemic, APNs were confronted with numerous tasks to stay current and at pace with rapid changes occurring in the health care environment, ultimately leading to substantial work-related stress. Based on self reported mental health and well-being from respondents within the health care workforce to the Behavioral Risk Factor Surveillance System (BRFSS) from 2017–2019, insufficient sleep (41%) and diagnosed depression (19%) were the two most frequently reported conditions (Silver et al., 2022). The strains felt by APNs were evident, yet APNs sustained a vigorous energy toward positive influences on health care delivery and reform.

APN Clinician

In the few years prior to the onset of the pandemic, the APN clinician was finding momentum as primary care providers and leading the charge as change agents. A *change agent* is defined by Rogers (2010) as people who introduce innovations into a client system that they expect will have consequences that will be desirable, direct, and anticipated. This definition will play a key underpinning to the proposed framework for nursing theory as a tool for the APN in the post-pandemic era.

With this momentum, 28 states and the District of Columbia have adopted full practice authority for nurse practitioners, enabling them to perform practice without the supervision or collaboration with a physician. The expansion of NP practice authority was positively received as a means to address a growing physician shortage and a means to lower costs. A trend in altering the roles of the APN clinician can be summarized by Blumenthal and Abrams in 2013 as five guiding principles for U.S. health care policy in the future: policy reform reflecting professional competencies and not long-standing state laws; policies being dynamic and responsive to evolving roles, organization, and financing health care; incorporating patient preferences about receiving primary care services; rebuilding the primary care infrastructure; and collaboration between NPs and physicians to improve delivery of primary care. A movement was in place to develop interdisciplinary care frameworks that addressed education, practice, policy and evaluation for all APNs, physicians, and physician assistants.

To illustrate the efforts of the APN clinician's positive impacts on health care, studies were performed to raise awareness through quantitative measures of NPs' value in health outcomes and financial viability. A retrospective study of 30 million patient visits to community health centers found that NPs cared for similar patient populations as physicians and achieved equivalent or better results on quality metrics, such as depression treatment, physical exams, medication use, return visits, and referrals (Kurtzman & Barnow, 2017). In addition, a financial impact was identified; using Medicare claims, patients managed by NPs cost 29% less than patients managed by physicians, even after adjusting for comorbidities (Perloff et al., 2016). Despite promising studies, more research was projected to assess the financial implications of NP practice. Needless to say, APN clinicians were expanding and producing positive effects on health care.

Nurse Practitioner Practice Authority: A State-by-State Guide

For more information on full practice, reduced practice, and restricted practice for nurse practitioners, please visit the link provided:

- https://nursejournal.org/nurse-practitioner/np-practice-authority-by-state/

APN Leader

Prior to the pandemic, APN leaders were strengthening their course to influence policy and politics to fund health care systems and socioeconomic policies affecting communities' health. A major driver for the APN leader was demonstrated globally in the purposeful awareness of the Sustainable Development Goals (SDGs). APN leaders recognized the importance of cross-sectoral policy work and collaboration to make an operational imprint on shaping nursing's response to health issues on a practice level at local, regional, national, and global health stages. APN leaders engaged in active roles to influence and lead policy changes and development. In this process, APN leaders took aim to drive policy while understanding the context or need for change and sharing critical information with health care stakeholders. Change agents became synonymous with the APN leader.

United Nations Department of Economic and Social Affairs/Sustainable Development

For more information on the SDGs, visit the following link:

- https://sdgs.un.org/goals

Despite APN leaders work in policy development, change was slow. More was needed from nurse leaders to keep stride with the demands of health care in the years before the pandemic. Nursing recognized to have a prevailing voice at all levels of health and policy systems, it would require broader support than what was available from within nursing professional organizations (Salvage & White, 2019). As mentioned earlier in the chapter, VBC was a prevailing agenda for health care reform. Nurse leaders were placed in pivotal positions to lead health care toward a VBC system.

Nurse leaders are paramount in driving the transformation of the nation's health system to one that is value-based, achieves preferred outcomes, and focuses on improving health and quality care (National Advisory Council on Nurses, 2019). Based on the report by the National Advisory Council on Nurses (2019), APNs serve roles in multiple settings and in numbers alone can serve as leaders in the transformation of health care from volume based to value based. To answer this need and call to lead change to VBC, APN leaders initiated a focus on team-based care. In these efforts APN leaders and other influential members from the National Advisory Council on Nursing Education and Practice (NACNEP) called for an emphasis to be placed on VBC and team-based care in education, training, and licensure to provide high-quality, cost-effective care. Even through evaluations of efforts completed since the landmark report by the IOM (2011, now the National Academy of Medicine), *The Future of Nursing Report*, gaps were identified, and more needed to be done to integrate team-based care models into patient and family care processes (National Advisory Council on Nurses, 2019).

As APN leaders strived to be change agents in VBC and team-based care collaborations, nursing voices needed to be stronger and louder to ensure nurses are working to their full scope of practice. As mentioned earlier in the book, Magnet hospitals are recognized by the American Nurses Credentialing Center as performing better on value-based measures, higher patient satisfaction rates, and greater performance on value-based measurement (Lasater et al., 2016). During the decade before the pandemic, APN leaders strived to make the change to VBC and team-based care knowing nursing's voice and leadership skills could change the path of health care systems to adopt holistic and value-based practices, policies, and standards of care.

APN Educator

Nursing has had significant changes to practice as well as educational preparations in the past few decades, as illustrated in Chapters 1 and 2. As discussed with challenges of health care reform and the shifting landscape of the nursing workforce, nursing education has had to be proactive in integrating concepts, such as team-based nursing, into curricula. The APN educator not only adapts to changing demographics of students, but also learns new pedagogies and remains current in all aspects of health care delivery and reform.

Increased education preparation has made noteworthy impacts on health outcomes and influenced the call for higher education among nurses. In 2003, a study published in the *Journal of the American Medical Association* found a 10% increase in the number of BSN-prepared nurses reduced the likelihood of patient death by 5% (Aiken et al., 2003). As the statistics suggest, the promise of improved patient outcomes and the simultaneous cost savings created a flurry of interest from health care system leaders and stakeholders. Organizations and stakeholders inferred potential outcomes of employing BSN-prepared nurses, including lower turnover costs, a stable workforce, lower mortality rates, safer practice environments, and a more prepared pipeline of well-prepared nursing staff to fill management and leadership roles. All items would greatly impact a VBC system toward improved health outcomes.

One of the biggest calls on APN educators is to be active in the recruitment of nurses to complete higher education preparations. In 2009, the Carnegie Foundation released *Educating Nurses: A Call for Radical Transformation*, arguing that schools and the profession must take drastic steps to keep pace with rapid changes in health care (Benner, 2012). Part of the report from the then IOM called for nurses to achieve higher levels of education and training through an improved education system that promotes seamless progression. At the time, 3 million nurses were the single largest segment of the health care workforce. The AARP Foundation and the Robert Wood Johnson Foundation created initiatives to carry out the IOM's report. A major goal was to urge 80% of all practicing nurses to earn or have earned a bachelor's degree by the year 2020. By May of 2010, the Tri-Council for Nursing, which included the American Association of Colleges of Nursing, the ANA, the American Organization of Nurse Executives (AONE), and the National League for Nursing, issued a statement encouraging all nurses, regardless of entry point into the profession, to continue their education in programs that grant baccalaureate, master's, and doctoral degrees. By 2016, the number of RNs who obtained a bachelor's in nursing increased by 60,000 since 2010 (Benner, 2012).

Other influences, such as the passage of the ACA in 2010, the drive for full extent of scopes of practice, and the need for nurse leaders, made substantial impacts on nursing education. APN educators were called to be fluid in their curriculum design and implementation to address numerous demands for the practicing nurse. To ensure sufficient and effective integration of health care trends, five education models were supported to promote seamless academic progression for actively working RNs. In addition to the five education models, APN educators collaborated and developed strong partnerships with community colleges and universities to cover broad geographical areas, hold national professional accreditation and institutional accreditation, work in conjunction with financial aid partners, increase the diversity of the nursing workforce, and encourage nurses to seek work in rural areas. APN educators were rising to the challenge to meet the demands of health care and to prepare future nurses at all levels to practice safely and efficiently in VBC health-led environments.

Five education models were widely adopted to support nursing education to be more fluid in addressing complexities in health situations and to ensure students do not meet unnecessary roadblocks when seeking higher academic preparation. (Note: All models listed are based on the AACN's "Essentials of Baccalaureate Education for Professional Nursing Practice.")

- outcomes- or competency-based curriculum
- curriculum shared at the state or regional level
- RN-to-BSN degree from a community college
- dual admission/dual enrollment
- accelerated options for RN to MSN

APN Role Transitions Amid a Pandemic

COVID-19 changed the health care landscape on a global level. How people work, socialize, and learn changed to the extent that previous cultures of social interaction on personal and professional levels were altered. The role of the nurse drastically changed to a sense of personal responsibility. As the pandemic intersected more and more communities and the resources to care for patients, nursing voices became louder. Nurses assumed the bulk of care and exposure to dangers on a worldwide scale. Due to the need for nurses, many states and the federal government promoted an increase in nurse flexibility. Since the pandemic, the realization of the changing roles of the nurse and APN have remained a priority topic in policy debates among state boards and medical associations, which are seeing a tip in the scale toward increasing nursing's scopes of practice. A real opportunity is presented post-pandemic for nurses to voice their changing roles and be recognized for their growing contributions to health care delivery.

The pandemic brought five distinct challenges to health care systems nationally: remote care, increasing health care costs, poor patient outcomes, health care disparities, and ethical challenges. The pandemic proved the health care system, despite its enormity, had to change quickly, out of necessity. More people paused and reflected on their individual health and what it meant to be well and healthy. Health care providers were beginning to understand interdisciplinary collaboration was more than a model of care but a necessity to provide both access to care and meet patients' needs. From a systems level, the pandemic highlighted inequities from multiple avenues, such as access to care and cost of coverage, creating a need for health care leaders to focus in depth on a supply and demand cycle to evaluate what is needed in health care and what needs to change.

Remote Care

One example that stands out from the pre-pandemic changes to health care is the use of technology to provide remote care. Telemedicine had limited use in health care pre-pandemic due to restrictions with payor payment and minimal evidence on its efficacy. Since COVID-19, telemedicine has become increasingly accessible beyond rural locations. With the CDC recommendations of social distancing, utilization of telemedicine climbed sharply. A 154% increase in telemedicine visits occurred in the last week of March 2020 than did in the same period in 2019 (Koonin et al., 2020). Because of the pandemic, telemedicine was relatively widely accepted by patients and clinicians (Almathami et al., 2020). Despite this increase in digital use, challenges emerged or were heightened.

Limited access to the internet or smart devices raised an inequity known as the digital divide. However, those who choose not to use telehealth services are not to be misrepresented as disconnected or slow to adopt to all offerings of technology. In evaluation and alignment of some of the largest users of health care, it is essential to acknowledge 86% of the more than 70 million Americans on Medicaid own a smartphone (Majerol & Carroll, 2018). According to Fitzpatrick et al. (2021), young Americans of color and underserved communities have used digital technology for health care; however, older people or those with lower digital literacy do not have tailored solutions to enhance their digital use. APNs can be champions to assuring access to health care through the use of digital health technologies. With respect to digital health technology, patient care saw an unlimited access to patient portals since the pandemic. The use of instant messaging has increased between patients and their primary health care providers, with less patients seeking specialty care, potentially demonstrating patient changes in how they would like to seek health care. At the heart of the health care environment remains the need to provide safe, quality care for patients. APNs in all roles can be catalysts to this requirement and influence policy and practice through innovation.

High Health Care Costs

To say the pandemic made a financial explosion on the U.S. health care system is to say the earth is round. Since the onset of COVID-19, a reported 80 million COVID cases, nearly 1 million deaths, and over 4.6 million hospitalizations stamped a substantial toll on health systems across the nation (Johns Hopkins Coronavirus Resource Center, n.d.). Health care systems were driven to be agile to react to the health crisis by hiring more staff,

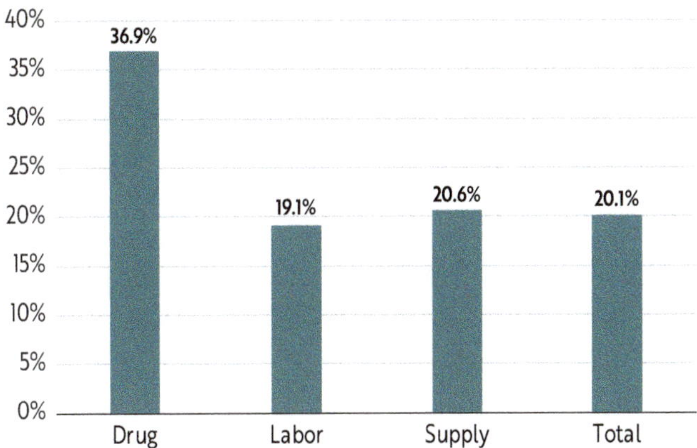

FIGURE 4.1 Increase in hospital expenses per patient from 2019 to 2021.

acquiring supplies, and expanding treatment capacities. To gain the most fair and accurate insight into the cost of the pandemic on health care systems, a broad view is required. Some of the most pressing punches to health care budgets were the increasing complexity of patients with intensifying effects on preexisting co-morbidities, zero government assistance through the COVID-19 Provider Relief Fund (PRF) during the delta and omicron variant surges, loss of staff (including a nursing exodus), inflation (economy wide and medical supply costs), Medicare cuts, inpatient payment rate for Medicare patients, and rising hospital labor costs, all which dramatically affected increases in health care costs (Swanson, 2022).

In assessing the high cost of health care, a view of the public's experiences with health care costs needs to be presented. According to the Kaiser Family Foundation's data note, the following public perceptions on health care costs have been identified:

- About half of U.S. adults say they have difficulty affording health care costs.
- Substantial shares of adults 65 or older report difficulty paying for various aspects of health care, especially services not generally covered by Medicare, such as hearing services and dental and prescription drug costs.
- The cost of health care often prevents people from getting needed care or filling prescriptions. About a quarter of adults say they or family member in their household have not filled a prescription, cut pills in half, or skipped doses of medicine in the last year because of the cost, with larger shares of those in households with lower incomes, Black and Hispanic adults, and women reporting this.
- High health care costs disproportionately affect uninsured adults, Black and Hispanic adults, and those with lower incomes. Larger shares of U.S. adults in each of these groups report difficulty affording various types of care and delaying or forgoing medical care due to the cost.
- Those who are covered by health insurance are not immune to the burden of health care costs. About one third of insured adults worry about affording their monthly health insurance premium, and 44% worry about affording their deductible before health insurance kicks in.
- Health care debt is a burden for a large share of Americans. About four in 10 adults (41%) report having debt due to medical or dental bills, including debts owed to credit cards, collections agencies, family and friends, banks, and other lenders to pay for their health care costs,

with disproportionate shares of Black and Hispanic adults, women, parents, those with low incomes, and uninsured adults saying they have health care debt.

- Affording gasoline and transportation costs is now a top worry for Americans followed by unexpected medical bills. While worry over gasoline and transportation costs has risen markedly since 2020, significant shares of adults still say they are worried about affording medical costs such as unexpected bills, deductibles, and long-term care services for themselves or a family member (Lopes et al., 2022).

As APNs are at the forefront of patient care and assessing patient needs, it is critically important for them to lead innovative change to prevent a decline in overall patient outcomes. The pandemic created fear, leading to an increase in people not seeking health care or delaying needed care. The impact of the public's worry to carry the burden of rising health care costs or debt can be detrimental to public health and impart continuous soaring of costs. Many patients have looming worries over covering household expenses, such as food, gasoline, heat, water, and rent or mortgage. Health care needs tend to be delayed to paying everyday living costs. In 2020, out-of-pocket and private insurance spending declined for the first time in recorded history, but overall health spending in the United States grew with the added effect from federal relief (Cox et al., 2021). Hospitals are now required to provide price transparency online, yet one in 10 adults are aware of this change (Cox et al., 2021). As the solutions to rising health care costs need a multi-level approach, which includes public awareness, the APN can be a partner to create innovation at the point of care, generating policy decisions and designing curriculum and learning strategies to ensure appropriate, efficient, safe, and evidence-based care and education is provided to all health care partners (nurses, physicians, patients, and students).

Poor Patient Outcomes

As has been described in the rising costs of health care and in the effects of delayed care, patient outcomes become a top concern for the APN. Furthermore, VBC can only be measured by quality, and this relates to what matters most to patients. Nevertheless, how are outcomes measures defined? According to the WHO (n.d.b.) an outcome measure is a change in the health of an individual, group of people, or population that is attributable to an intervention or series of interventions. To health care–associated systems, these are specific targets based on quality and cost, which each organization is continuously trying to improve.

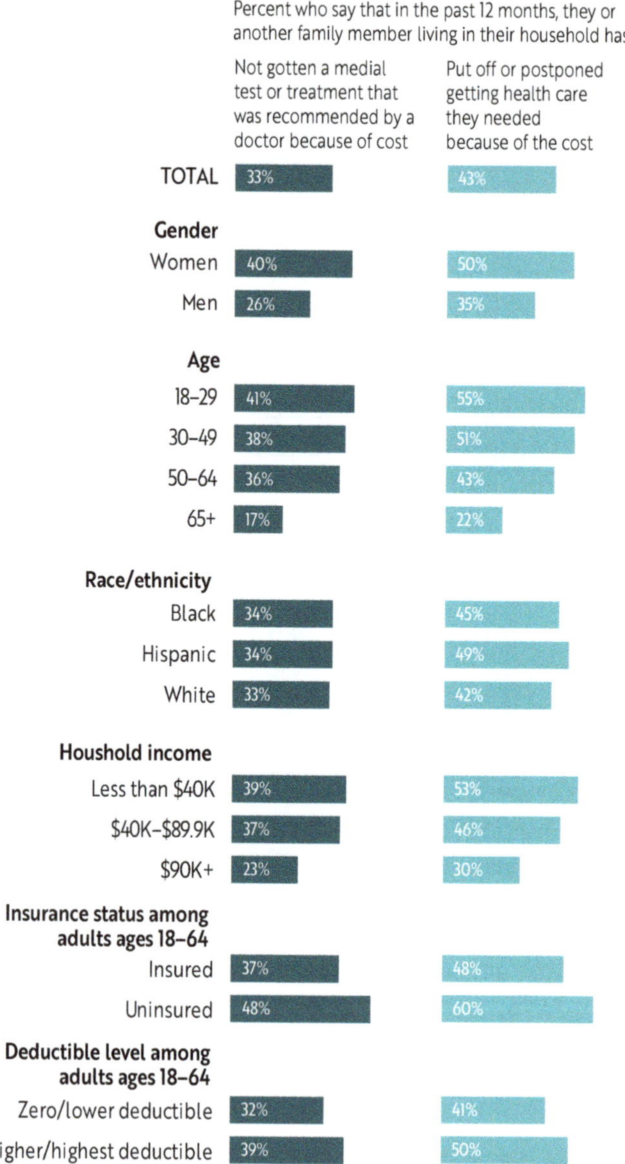

FIGURE 4.2 One third of adults say they or a family member have skipped recommended medical treatment due to cost, while four in 10 say they have delayed needed care.

Outcome measures can include metrics such as (a) mortality rates, (b) readmissions, (c) safety of care, (d) effectiveness of care, (e) patient experience, (f) timeliness of care, and (g) efficient use of medical imaging. Most of these target areas are reported to the federal government, commercial payers, and organizations, which specifically report on quality to provide transparency among health care providers. It is important for the APN to understand outcome measures are driven by national standards and financial incentives.

TABLE 4.1 National Organizations Who Define and Prioritize National Standards

Organization	Organization's Mission	Relation to National Standards (Patient Outcomes)	Organizational Link
Centers for Medicare and Medicaid Services (CMS)	The CMS (n.d.) Office of Minority Health (OMH) will lead the advancement and integration of health equity in the development; evaluation; and implementation of CMS's policies, programs, and partnerships.	CMS grouped outcome measures into seven categories weighted by importance: • Mortality (22%) • Safety of care (22%) • Readmissions (22%) • Patient experience (22%) • Effectiveness of care (4%) • Timeliness of care (4%) • Efficient use of medical imaging (4%)	Home - Centers for Medicare & Medicaid Services | CMS. (n.d.). https://www.cms.gov/
Joint Commission	Continuously improve health care for the public, in collaboration with other stakeholders, by evaluating health care organizations and inspiring them to excel in providing safe and effective care of the highest quality and value (Joint Commission, n.d.).	• Relate to patient safety or quality of care. • Positively impact health care outcomes. • Meet or surpass law and regulation. • Accurately and readily measure.	The Joint Commission. (n.d.). A trusted partner in patient care. https://www.jointcommission.org/
National Association for Healthcare Quality (NAHQ)	To prepare a coordinated, competent workforce to lead and advance healthcare quality across the continuum of healthcare (NAHQ, n.d.).	Develops health care quality competencies offering NAHQ education, certification, and networking.	NAHQ - National Association for Healthcare Quality. (n.d.). NAHQ. https://nahq.org/

A direct relationship to poor patient outcomes as a result of the pandemic can be linked to less patients using preventative screenings and treatments, such as vaccinations. Children missed or were placed on delayed schedules for routine childhood vaccines. Meanwhile a 90% drop in cancer screenings occurred, delaying diagnoses and subsequent treatments (Koonin et al., 2020). With surveys from organizations such as the Kaiser Family Foundation, public fear during the pandemic has created a sequelae of events that will provide continued effects on life expectancy and medical needs associated with chronic care management.

Health Care Disparities

The pandemic has led to high stress effecting the physical, emotional, and mental well-being for many Americans. The effects of COVID-19 shifted referrals from medical needs to referrals for items such as housing, food access, and supplemental income, resulting in a wider understanding of health care disparities. During and since the COVID-19 pandemic, health disparities have been largely unmasked. The pandemic revealed a disproportionate effect of COVID-19 infections across the nation, and these were higher among certain ethnic groups. The Centers for Disease Control and Prevention (CDC) tracked COVID-19 testing, vaccination rates, hospitalizations, and deaths, which showed a 2.8 times higher mortality rate of Indian/Alaska Native people dying from COVID-19 than White people with age considered (U.S. Government Accountability Office, n.d.). For the APN, it is essential to understand the relationship that exists between patient outcomes and patients with health disparities. For example, the following identified health disparities highlight specific patient outcomes:

- *COVID-19.* Available data show that between March 2020 and June 2021, Hispanic or Latino and non-Hispanic Black people were hospitalized with COVID-19 at a rate 2.8 times higher than non-Hispanic White people, when taking age into account.
- *Pregnancy-related deaths.* From 2011–2016, Black women living in rural counties experienced 59.3 deaths per 100,000 live births compared to 19.7 for White women in the same counties, according to CDC data.
- *Life expectancy and chronic health conditions.* In 2018, the diabetes age-adjusted mortality rate was higher among Black people (49.7 deaths per 100,000 people) and American Indian/Alaska Native people (40.0 deaths) than White people (24.8 deaths).
- *Veterans' health.* Black veterans with cancer and cardiovascular-related illnesses had lower survival rates than White veterans (U.S. Government Accountability Office, n.d.).

As the APN understands health disparities on a broader scale and considers root causes such as socioeconomic status, age, geography, language, gender, disability status, citizenship status, and sexual identity and orientation, APNs can apply priority assessments to identify health disparities. Higher rates of illness and death among certain ethnic groups can reflect increased exposures of bacterial and viral infections due to living, working, and transportation circumstances alongside preexisting health conditions. APNs can serve to be solution makers for health disparities by considering broader implications, such as social justice, equity, and overall national health and economic prosperity.

Ethical Challenges

The pandemic unveiled numerous ethical challenges in all health care settings. Health care providers were confronted with triage decisions, shortages of key resources, visitor restrictions, quality care (limitations/short staffing), and end-of-life decisions without a family/social support presence. All health care providers made ethical decisions while maintaining professional duties. In turn, health care providers experienced extreme levels of psychological trauma and moral distress. *Burnout*, defined as a state of fatigue or frustration that results in a professional relationship that failed to produce expected rewards, can be further applied to the nurse during and after the pandemic (Sullivan et al., 2021). All of these factors can be linked to nurse turnover,

TABLE 4.2 APN Roles: Responses to the Five Post-Pandemic Impacts

Post-Pandemic Impacts	APN Clinician	APN Leader	APN Educator
Remote Care (Telehealth/ Telemedicine)	Health care provided via technology should be recognized, regulated, and reimbursed on parity with the same services delivered in person. AANP endorses the use of the term telehealth to refer to these services.	Nurse leaders play a critical role in the successful implementation and practice of telehealth nursing. They may help develop protocols for its use and assist in acquiring or establishing equipment. They also are responsible for motivating nursing staff to embrace telehealth by emphasizing its benefits for both nurses and patients.	Many nursing programs do not equip nurses with adequate telehealth instruction, and graduates enter the workforce without the necessary competencies and skills. Because of this gap in learning, nurse educators will play a key role in modernizing nurse education programs and readying nurses for the rise in telehealth services.

(Continued)

TABLE 4.2 APN Roles: Responses to the Five Post-Pandemic Impacts (*Continued*)

Post-Pandemic Impacts	APN Clinician	APN Leader	APN Educator
High Health Care Costs	NPs are a proven response to the evolving trend toward wellness and preventive health care driven by consumer demand. A solid body of evidence demonstrates that NPs have consistently proven to be cost-effective providers of high-quality care.	Nurse leaders work directly within the triple aim framework (the Institute of Healthcare Improvement) by optimizing care in population health, experience of care, and cost of providing that care.	Nurse educators are instrumental in shaping the future of the nursing profession, encouraging a focus on holistic patient care and illness prevention to reduce healthcare costs.
Poor Patient Outcomes	Research has found that patients under the care of NPs have fewer unnecessary hospital readmissions, fewer potentially preventable hospitalizations, higher patient satisfaction, and fewer unnecessary emergency room visits than patients under the care of physicians.	Nurse leaders oversee a team of nurses, making decisions and directing patient care initiatives. They have advanced clinical knowledge and are focused on improving patient health outcomes.	Nurse educators motivate and educate students and staff to adopt new practice changes, incorporating evidence-based practices that promote positive patient outcomes.
Health Care Disparities	APN clinicians get more face time with patients, which puts nurses in a position to uncover certain SDOH.	Nurse leaders create change in their institutions and therefore can advocate for reduced health disparities.	Nurse educators play a special role in ensuring that students can identify SDOH and participate in developing and implementing strategies to reduce health disparities for individuals, groups, and populations.

TABLE 4.2 APN Roles: Responses to the Five Post-Pandemic Impacts (*Continued*)

Post-Pandemic Impacts	APN Clinician	APN Leader	APN Educator
Ethical Challenges	APN clinicians must be able to recognize ethical conflicts and serve as mediators or resources for patients, families, or other nurses who struggle with ethical dilemmas.	Nurse leaders have a pivotal role in balancing the care of their staff with the care of the patients they serve. As critical members of the executive team, nurse leaders represent and give voice to frontline ethical challenges.	Nurse educators have the responsibility of assisting students and their colleagues with understanding and practicing ethical conduct.

or the voluntary and early termination of nurses' employment. As nursing shortages continue to increase, a sequelae of ethical challenges will persist.

Other ethical dilemmas identified as a result of the pandemic can be viewed as extensions of health care costs, health disparities, and socioeconomic factors. For example, intimate partner violence (IPV) became a major public health crisis nationally and worldwide during the period of lockdowns and social distancing protocols. APNs can include in their roles ways to address IPV and apply real-time solutions through medical interventions, social support referrals, and education (awareness). Ethical challenges are a mainstay in an environment like health care; however, the APN can make persistent strides in educating others about ethical principles and adhering to ethical codes.

APN Post-Pandemic Health Care Opportunities: Invigorating Innovation

The pandemic made long-lasting impacts on health care, yet the outlook can be positive and should be seen as an opportunity. While APNs reflect and give honor to all those who lost their lives to COVID-19, they can also channel innovation toward value-based health care, which views "value" in a new way. As leaders in nursing who are intimately aware of the needs of patients, there is a natural proclivity for APNs to bring mindfulness to health care systems toward building healthier and more sustainable health care offerings. By understanding the challenges facing health care, APNs can become change agents by working toward a cultural shift for strengthening and revisioning characteristics of VBC. These characteristics can be summarized by the author of *Care After Covid: What the Pandemic Revealed Is Broken in Healthcare and How to Reinvent It* as the following concepts: connectivity, distributed care, and digitally enabled care (Nundy, 2021).

Connectivity

Connectivity has taken on new meaning in health care since the onset of the pandemic. With the swift adjustments to telemedicine, health care providers used technology to "see" patients and respond to their emergent needs. Connectivity can be exemplified in establishing authenticity with patient encounters and relationships, and connectivity can be used for addressing patient outreach in innovative ways to ensure patients have accessible and VBC. APNs are keenly aware and agents of establishing therapeutic relationships with patients. The essential attributes of relationships between nurses and patients are empathy, presence, contact, authenticity, trust, and reciprocity (Allande-Cussó et al., 2021). The "value" of establishing effective and satisfying relationships with patients is critical to patient outcomes.

Example of Connectivity and Collaboration With a Nurse Practitioner–Driven Program to Positively Affect Patient Outcomes

In a study conducted over 2 years by a New England–managed care organization with a large Medicaid membership, a comprehensive primary care model was offered in the homes of patients with complex, medical, social, and behavioral conditions known as the Health@Home program (Trilla et al., 2018). Health@Home is a team-based program led by nurse practitioners to evaluate the short- and long-term effects of reducing rates and associated costs of medical and behavioral health inpatient hospital admission and emergency departments by providing intensive, high-touch interventions in the patient's home (Trilla et al., 2018). The program goals were to develop patient-centered care with reengagement with patients and their primary care providers (Trilla et al., 2018). The NPs worked collaboratively with interdisciplinary members to perform patient assessments and to identify a risk assessment to ensure effective allocation of resources were utilized. Medical inpatient admits per 1,000 decreased 39.2% from baseline 1 to intervention and continued to decrease an additional 29.9% in the 2 years after the intervention, for a total reduction of 57.4% from baseline 1 to year 2 post (Trilla et al., 2018). In addition, costs over the length of the program showed immediate and long-term declines in total medical expenses (Trilla et al., 2018). NPs demonstrated a program intervention whereby not only was a collaborative framework utilized, but the program allowed for the NP to work intimately with the patient in their home and create a connectivity to the patient, resulting in financial improvements and overall health-improved outcomes for participants.

Distributed Care

Nundy (2021) describes distributed care as the notion care should happen where health happens, at home and in the community. Wherever patients are should be where APNs can reimagine offering care services. Nundy reminds health care providers that delivering health care where patients live and work can better address root causes of poor health. Eighty-eight percent of NPs certified in primary care, and 70% of all NPs deliver primary care (AANP, n.d.). The opportunity for APN clinicians to offer solutions and methods to implement distributed care is extensive. Ideas on the horizon for distributed care can include the following:

- Virtual care: Real-time telehealth monitoring
- Mobile care: Health care providers come to the patient
- Walk-in care: Expansion of clinics at stores
- New hospital patients: Can seek specialized care while in hospital (Philips, n.d.).

Philips Future Health Index Report (2022)

Health care leaders now view extending care delivery beyond the hospital as their highest priority after staff satisfaction and retention (Philips, n.d.). A key finding of the Philips study is that 40% of hospitals are expecting to shift about 20% of their cases to patients' homes by 2025 (Philips, n.d.).

Digitally Enabled Care

Digitally enabled care refers to using the right role of technology in health care to increase care (Nundy, 2021). The interest for virtual care platforms has increased and sustained since the pandemic for both health care providers and patients. The AMA studied the value of digitally enabled care on a wide range of virtual care programs in increasing overall health for patients, clinicians, payors, and the society. In the AMA's (2022) research, known as the "Return on Health" framework, six value streams were used with specific metrics to capture value in virtual care programs:

- clinical outcomes, quality, and safety
- access to care
- patient, family, and caregiver experience
- clinician experience

- financial and operational impact
- health equity

The framework can be used by APN leaders to develop and evaluate new models of care and policies to support accessible, quality-driven, and affordable virtual care services.

APNs are uniquely positioned as clinicians, leaders, and educators to address the Institute of Healthcare Improvement's (n.d.) triple aim, which calls for health care professionals to deliver care with an emphasis on improving patient quality and satisfaction, improve overall population health, and reduce the cost of health care. Specific skill sets will be required to assist the APN in their unique role to use tools, such as nursing theory, to guide practice, policy, and learning.

TABLE 4.3 APN Attributes to Positively Invigorate Health Care Innovation

VBC Innovation	APN Clinician	APN Leader	APN Educator
Connectivity	· Authentic communication · Altruistic presence · Empathy · Advocate · Embracer of diversity	· Proactive · Precise communication · Negotiator · Professional socialization · Emotional intelligence	· Inspirational · Patience · Natural curiosity
Distributed Care	· Flexible practice · Autonomous · Collaborator · Competence · Service oriented	· Coordinator · Policymaker · Financially conscious · Promoter of employee development · Pioneer	· Clinical knowledge of health care delivery trends · Forward thinking to design education
Digitally Enabled Care	· Resourceful · Ethically conscious · Active listener · Intuitive	· Detail oriented · Technologically proficient	· Continual learner · Technologically savvy to integrate technology applications in education

Figure Credits

Fig. 4.1: American Hospital Association, "Increase in Hospital Expenses Per Patient from 2019 to 2021," https://www.aha.org/guidesreports/2023-04-20-2022-costs-caring. Copyright © 2022 by American Hospital Association.

Fig. 4.2: KFF, "One-Third of Adults Say They or a Family Member Have Skipped Recommended Medical Treatment Due to Cost, While Four in Ten Say They Have Delayed Needed Care," https://www.kff.org/health-costs/issue-brief/americans-challenges-with-health-care-costs/. Copyright © 2023 by KFF.

CHAPTER 5

Metacognition's Relationship to Theory-Guided Practice

Key Terms

AI: A branch of computer science that attempts to both understand and build intelligent entities, often instantiated as software programs (Yu et al., 2018).

Concept: A psychological endowment that organizes one's knowledge and underpins human reasoning (Shea, 2019).

Internet of Things (IoT): An extended and expanded system network based on the internet and its ultimate goal to achieve real-time interaction among things, machines, and humans through various advanced technological means (Wang et al., 2021).

Metacognition: "Thinking about thinking" (Dunlosky & Metcalfe, 2008).

Nursing concept(s): Include central themes represented in the metaparadigm: person, health, nurse, and environment.

Reflective practice: A cognitive skill that demands conscious effort to look at a situation with an awareness of one's beliefs, values, and practice, enabling nurses to learn from experiences and incorporate that learning in improving patient care outcomes (Patel & Metersky, 2021).

Introduction

Influences such as the pandemic, the retirement of the baby boomer generation, and changing health care delivery platforms have shaped specific nursing trends the profession will need to stay abreast of and be innovative in its response. The growth rate of advanced practice jobs in relation to supply and demand will continue to increase. The U.S. Bureau of Labor Statistics (2022) projects a job growth rate of 45% for APNs by 2030. With the demand for APNs increasing at a fast pace, APNs can charge new ideas to health care delivery standards and policies through proactive responses.

TABLE 5.1 Health Care Trends and APN Proactive Response(s)

Health Care/Nursing Trend	APN Proactive Response
Home health will increase in popularity and usage.	*APN clinician*: Home health can be a lifeline for vulnerable populations, creating an opportunity for APN clinicians to lead the charge in home care with the implementation of telehealth services and skilled practitioners to set safe, quality standardizations of care and optimal use of resources.
Care models will experience a more flexible shift.	*APN leader*: Team-based nursing can be an innovative and flexible model for an increasingly complex patient population while ensuring competent skill sets are present to deliver required care.
Training and higher education will be in demand.	*APN educator*: The AACN (n.d.c.) promotes the preference of nurses who hold a Bachelor of Science in nursing (BSN) with about 82% of employers expressing a strong preference for BSN-prepared nurses. APN educators will be in demand to prepare nurses in formative and incentive-based programs.

As part of this journey to 2030, APNs and nurses alike can use tools to assist in their adaptability and knowledge growth within the changing clinical and nonclinical health care environments. As APNs and nurses feel the weight of personal responsibility to their patients, staff, and students while constantly maneuvering to adjust to shifting health care trends and standards, retaining new knowledge and skills can become overwhelming and feel futile. Prior to adopting theory-guided practice as a skill set, with theory used as tools to advance practice, the APN can use methods to comprehend their maturing knowledge and commitment to leading health care to a value-, evidenced-, and patient-centered care model.

The chapter will address the following learning objectives:

1. Discover metacognition as a skill set for the advanced practice nurse to assist in adapting to new health care environments and lead the charge to innovative health care practices.
2. Distinguish metacognition as a unique tool to assist each APN role of clinician, leader, and educator in effective and efficient role development in the post-pandemic era.
3. Construct a metacognition philosophy as a positive action toward a "reflect-in-practice" viewpoint.

What Is Metacognition?

Prior to dissecting metacognition, it is important for the APN to comprehend the term *concept*. Concepts are described by Shea (2019) as tools for thinking, such as categorization, learning, induction, and action planning, used as mental representations during conscious deliberate thought. Nursing theory is immersed in nursing concepts. Nursing concepts are centralized around the metaparadigm, which include four distinct domains: person, nurse, health, and environment. Nursing utilizes the metaparadigm in research and in practice to demonstrate a fluid relationship as a foundation for action and reflection (Bender, 2018). In essence, the metaparadigm extends an approach to confirm nursing practices holistically. Holistic practice is a major nursing principle by recognizing the influential nature of each domain.

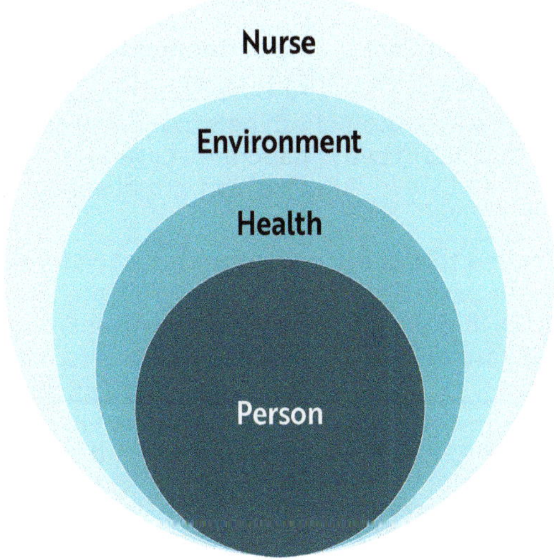

FIGURE 5.1 Nursing metaparadigm.

As nursing evolves and adapts to the changing health care landscape, the foundations of nursing theory and the domains of the metaparadigm remain constant; however, change can be recommended. To encourage dynamic nursing, change to the fundamentals found in theory and nursing frameworks can invigorate new ideas and research leading to safer, higher quality, and innovative care practices. For example, Johnson and Carrington (2023) propose the inclusion of technology as a concept to the nursing metaparadigm. By integrating technology as a domain of the nursing metaparadigm, nurses and APNs can seamlessly adapt to advanced technologies impacting patient care, leadership, and education. In addition, Johnson and Carrington suggest nursing science can advance to ensure patient-centered care remains a top priority to healthcare models and nursing practice.

Technology advancements, such as machine learning, allow AI to learn from surroundings to make intelligent decisions. The development of machine learning will affect patient care and influence new methods of practice for all health care providers. To illustrate the growth of AI, the total number of potential buyers in health care was $147.1 billion in 2018 and expected to increase by 19.9% each year (U.S. Bureau of Economic Analysis, n.d.). Technology and the Internet of Things (IoT) is present in health care, with demand soaring to develop methods to ensure value-driven care. In short, value-driven care seeks to link quality to payment. The value-driven movement includes health information technology as a priority in directing quality and price standards.

TABLE 5.2 AI Growth in Health Care and Opportunities for APNs

AI Expansion in U.S. Health Care	Opportunities for APNs
Artificial intelligence in the healthcare market grew at a rate of 167.1% from 2019 to 2021, in two years' time-period (Grand View Research, n.d.).	AI-based technologies in health care can be expanded into diagnostic tools, patient management, clinical trials, virtual care, and virtual education.
The market is estimated to witness a year-on-year growth range between 34.9% to 48.0% in the next 5 years (Grand View Research, n.d.).	APNs can be at the forefront of AI adoption by ensuring the technology can swiftly diagnose and detect underlying health conditions to meet the demands of an aging population with more chronic conditions while ensuring a value-based system provides the most effective and efficient care options.
Businesses are rapidly devising AI products to sell in an accelerated market with high competition.	APNs are critical in being part of the selection, assessment, evaluation, and adoption of AI technologies to ensure a nursing voice is integrated into care practices, care management, and education.

As concepts in nursing expand with the changes in health care trends and technology-based adoptions, nursing is centered in an era of flux, creating a need to use tools to prioritize, plan, organize, and implement the best care practices for patients, staff, and students. A tool commonly used in education can be highly valuable to the APN in this post-pandemic era: metacognition.

Metacognition is often defined as being able to evaluate and control one's own cognitive processes (Dunlosky & Metcalfe, 2008). Metacognition is believed to be a vital capacity with the implications for education, emotional regulation, and self-awareness (Dunlosky & Metcalfe, 2008). Metacognition is not merely memory, rather an individual judgment extending toward one's perceptions, resulting in shifting action performance. In the process of metacognition, a person builds confidence toward an action, thought process, and decision-making. Attributes that are invaluable skills to each APN role.

To adopt a broader understanding and application of metacognition, nursing can look to psychologists and philosophers' research in defining *metacognition* as a "set of capacities through which an operating subsystem is evaluated or represented by another subsystem in a context-sensitive way" (Proust, 2013, p. 4)—in other words, thinking about thinking. Bringing nursing insight to the concept of metacognition, Proust (2013) suggests metacognition represents an experience, a feeling, a perception, and action, leading to a sense of confidence. In further analysis, one can assume the act of metacognition leads to learning or knowing as defined by Carper's patterns of knowing.

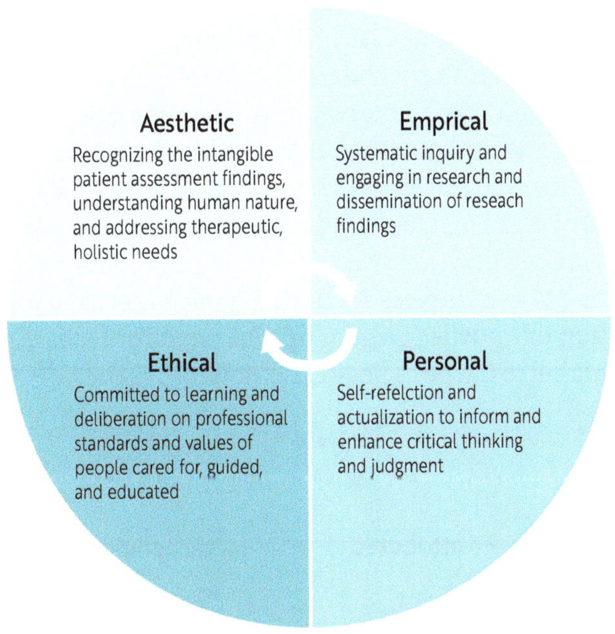

FIGURE 5.2 Carper's patterns of knowing and the APN.

Taking a Leap Beyond Reflective Practice

Metacognition, often referred to as reflection on action, has been used extensively in nursing education. It has served as a modality to enhance student perceptions and identification of new knowledge. As nurses begin to practice and throughout their careers, the skill of metacognition can be lost, unless the nurse reenters an academic program to advance their education and nursing practice. As nursing seeks sustenance in a post-pandemic era, skills, like metacognition, can provide support with a sense of confidence to address nursing practice concerns. With each new clinical and nonclinical setting issue, nurses are required to use effective reasoning and judgment. To be effective in reasoning and judgment, metacognitive skill acquisition is a necessary tool for nurses to adopt. Metacognition skill acquisition is accomplished through self-regulated, lifelong learning.

As nurses adapt practice and care interventions to meet patient needs and the demands of policies and care costs, metacognition skills can support them in recognizing what they know and what they do not know, hence making them a more effective and efficient care provider. Nurses can seek knowledge and information to fill the gaps of what they do not know, otherwise classified as self-regulated learning. A major element to effective self-regulated learning is understanding and practicing metacognition. *Metacognition* is the ability to monitor thinking, to use skills and strategies appropriately, and to achieve a desirable outcome.

Similar to metacognition is the concept of reflective practice. Reflective practice has been adopted in many professions, including medicine, education, business, and nursing (Patel & Metersky, 2021). Under the context of reflective practice, a cognitive skill is performed to review a situation with an awareness of one's own beliefs and practice (Patel & Metersky, 2021). Reflective practice allows for the nurse to engage in ongoing analysis by giving meaning to experiences and identifying patterns in practice, hence the recognition of knowledge gaps and/or need for research. Reflective practice is parallel to Carper's personal knowing, as the person engages in

Reflective practice attributes

- Integral to learning from experience (looking back)
- Directive process
- Enhance learning in the present
- Enhance personal experiences
- Identifies gaps in knowledge
- Recognizes cause and effect

Metacognition attributes

- Integral to learning from experience (looking ahead)
- Intrinsic motivation
- Growth mindset; lifelong learning
- Generate evidence and evolving knowledge
- Creates solutions
- Links knowing to doing

FIGURE 5.3 Enhancing reflective practice with metacognition.

reflection focused on learning through experiences. The act of reflecting is often perceived in a simplified manner and can lose its higher intent to connect theory and practice or knowing and doing. Under metacognition, as a lifelong, self-regulated skill set, the nurse and APN not only engage in a reflective process, but also consider innovation under the context of current trends and challenges faced in health care settings. In this process, the nurse and APN contemplate experiential learning, create a process to fill knowledge gaps, reconnect to nursing theory, and generate opportunities to address issues through innovation.

Advantages of Developing Metacognition Skills for the APN

As APNs have extensive backgrounds in practice, metacognition becomes more important to the adult learner through experiential learning modalities. Advanced degree students can benefit from metacognition processes by becoming increasingly aware of self-regulation and enhancing proficiencies in the learning process. The method of self-regulation permits the APN and student to recognize and appreciate individual strengths and weaknesses, resulting in learning and improvement. The act of metacognition can be carried into the APN's role and be a formidable skill set in using theory to guide practice, frame research, and continue to develop the nursing profession through innovative practice.

APNs are natural thinkers and learners. A caveat to being skilled in metacognition will require the APN to identify strengths and weaknesses. For the APN student and clinician, for example, this can be done by using assessment measures, such as the National Organization of Nurse Practitioner Faculties (NONPF, 2022) core competencies. To illustrate, domain 1, knowledge of practice, seeks the student and NP to integrate, translate, and apply established and evolving scientific knowledge from diverse sources as the basis for ethical clinical judgment, innovation, and diagnostic reasoning. Under this domain, a core competency is to apply theory and research-based knowledge from nursing. To continue to use this core competency, metacognition can be applied as a tool to address the student and NP's knowledge of theory and evidence to clinical practice (knowing to doing).

For the APN student and nurse leader, metacognition can be linked to emotional intelligence by fully understanding an event (issue) before acting. In this process of metacognition by the APN leader, a complete inventory of missing information is executed to identify next steps in a systematic approach. An APN leader can use metacognition to safeguard the least amount of bias to inform decision-making and advocacy for policy development constructed on critical analysis of the issue. Leadership theories can in tandem be used to guide metacognitive needs and future actions. Metacognition provides the APN student and leader the skills to avoid auto-pilot performance by highlighting the use of self-regulation to build confidence in leadership credentials.

For the APN student and educator, metacognition has been a traditional learning strategy in the classroom and clinical settings. APN educators have used metacognition, or reflective thinking, as exercises to enhance student clinical reasoning in promoting measures to safe practice. Nevertheless, the APN educator can benefit from adopting metacognition skills in their role. With the growing changes in the health care field, the APN educator must adapt pedagogies and learning strategies to meet the learning needs of students while also benefiting health care settings. This dual challenge for the APN educator calls for fluency and adaptability with a strong commitment to self-regulated learning, all attributes of the metacognition process.

The APN and Metacognition: Enhancing Role Effectiveness and Efficiency

One of the leading benefits of using metacognitive practice for the APN is improving the application of knowledge, skills, and professional role qualities to the real world. The APN has the tool and opportunity to make much-needed connections between theory and practice. Nursing theory-guided practice (NTGP) is focused on utilizing the assumptions set forth by theory to lead EBP interventions. Both EBP and NTGP are essential cogs in the APN's knowledge development wheel. As advanced nursing practice is underpinned by discipline-specific theoretical knowledge, metacognition creates a pathway to enlighten and remind the APN of the value of theory, research, and reflective practice. In the post-pandemic environment, it becomes essential for APNs to be collaborators of innovation while preserving nursing's exceptional contribution to health care.

For example, the use of metacognition allows the APN to transfer new knowledge, skills, and competencies to practice while interacting with other disciplines. Oftentimes in real-world settings, health care provider roles can become intersected with less clear-cut division of responsibilities. Adapting to changing situations (beyond what was learned in academic settings) is a challenge yet a necessity for the APN. This adaptation can be classified in the concept of transfer. Transfer of knowledge is a skill necessary to all professions, but it has an indispensable element for the APN.

The metacognition process provides direction for the APN to successfully transfer knowledge to practice. Key elements of the metacognition process include the following:

- knowing what you already know (general conceptual knowledge of a topic)
- desired knowledge (what do you want to learn)
- recognizing what you have learned (situational knowledge/Carper's patterns of knowing)
- selecting resources and learning strategies (planning to fill the knowledge gaps)
- monitoring new knowledge growth
- evaluating success of new knowledge growth (assessing usability of new knowledge to situational experiences for both present and future practice)

In addition to the proposed metacognition process for the APN, a final step in the process should promote inspirational thinking for the APN to address current and future issues to make positive and progressive impacts on health care and education. APNs can add creativity to practice by adding the final step of innovation. Promoting ingenuity to APN roles and practice can encourage the APN to fulfill the charge as trailblazers of health care.

As challenges in health care continue to prevail, APNs can use tools like metacognition to lead the changes needed to serve patients holistically with increased recognition of the impacts of SDOH. Social factors are incredibly influential in driving health consequences. The recognition of theses social factors can make the difference toward healthier and more satisfied outcomes for patients. A recent study suggests through health system innovation, improved health outcomes and reduced health care expenditures can occur (Pruitt et al., 2018). APNs can utilize resources such as Healthy People 2030, which has included social factors, such as food insecurity and insurance status, to guide patient interactions and individual assessments. To offer a demonstration of metacognition as a tool in addressing health disparities, a closer look is provided from the roles of APN clinician, leader, and educator.

Healthy People 2030

For more information on the leading health indicators addressed in Healthy People 2030, please use the following link:

- https://health.gov/healthypeople/objectives-and-data/leading-health-indicators

Metacognition Process for the APN in Addressing Health Disparities

TABLE 5.3 Metacognition Process: Transfer of Knowledge to Impact APN Clinician Role in Addressing Health Care Disparities

Metacognition Process/ Key Elements	APN Clinician	(#7) Proposed Final Step: Innovation Idea Starters
Knowing what you already know (general conceptual knowledge of a topic)	Being informed of health care disparities and their effects on patient outcomes	Decrease gaps in patient care access to resources by leading technology delivery models such as enhanced access to finding affordable prescriptions, offering telehealth rehabilitative therapy, and advocating for increased legislation to support primary care mobile health units.
Desired knowledge (what do you want to learn)	Effects of COVID-19 on health care access and use with vulnerable populations	
Recognizing what you have learned (situational knowledge/Carper's patterns of knowing)	Black and Hispanic patients have higher incidence to COVID-19 infections related to occupation and associated comorbidities	
Selecting resources and learning strategies (planning to fill the knowledge gaps)	Use of setting resources and knowledge of available resources to determine aligning SDOH	
Monitoring new knowledge growth	Applying assessment strategies for SDOH during all patient encounters	
Evaluating success of new knowledge growth (assessing usability of new knowledge to situational experiences for both present and future practice)	Employing evaluation techniques and critical patient follow-up to determine effectiveness and patient satisfaction	

TABLE 5.4 Metacognition Process: Transfer of Knowledge to Impact APN Leader Role in Addressing Health Care Disparities

Metacognition Process/ Key Elements	APN Leader	(#7) Proposed Final Step: Innovation Idea Starters
Knowing what you already know (general conceptual knowledge of a topic)	Being informed about health care disparities' impact on value-driven policies and standards of care	Expand nurse leadership competencies to include self-awareness tools and enhanced communication styles to achieve a shared vision and plan. Propose new value-based and equitable-centric policies to be integrated into organizational priorities at all levels of care, including technology applications.
Desired knowledge (what do you want to learn)	Seeking input from interdisciplinary leadership and state and federal legislation on policy development to enhance equity into new policies to lead value-based health care.	
Recognizing what you have learned (situational knowledge/Carper's patterns of knowing)	Using metacognition to review current or past situations when policy did not meet the standards of value-based and equitable care for all.	
Selecting resources and learning strategies (planning to fill the knowledge gaps)	Evaluating previous social health and system policies for congruence with VBC and equitable accountability.	
Monitoring new knowledge growth	Leading health care personnel to change with reenvisioned or newly developed policies with support and reaffirmation of system vision and mission goals.	
Evaluating success of new knowledge growth (assessing usability of new knowledge to situational experiences for both present and future practice)	Leading methods of strategic planning and evaluation of new policies to reflect a vision of inclusive and comprehensive health care.	

TABLE 5.5 Metacognition Process: Transfer of Knowledge to Impact APN Educator Role in Addressing Health Care Disparities

Metacognition Process/ Key Elements	APN Educator	(#7) Proposed Final Step: Innovation Idea Starters
Knowing what you already know (general conceptual knowledge of a topic)	Being informed on health care disparities and their role in educating students to assess for missed patient needs	Work with organizations such as the National League of Nursing to offer certification in health disparity education. Enhance simulation and technology-based educational programs to include SDOH in the clinical scenarios to enhance student understanding and application of SDOH assessment.
Desired knowledge (what do you want to learn)	Seeking current issues in health disparities and considering learning new approached to pedagogy, which enhances teaching of SDOH to students	
Recognizing what you have learned (situational knowledge/Carper's patterns of knowing)	Using metacognition to recognize clinical and educational settings which may have not upheld a standard of equitable care or lack of resources to ensure quality care is provided	
Selecting resources and learning strategies (planning to fill the knowledge gaps)	Pursuing continuing education for the nurse educator on SDOH and assessment strategies for students to identify patient needs and potential resources	
Monitoring new knowledge growth	Implementing new knowledge and competencies on culturally competent care and SDOH into curriculum and learning strategies	
Evaluating success of new knowledge growth (assessing usability of new knowledge to situational experiences for both present and future practice)	Using specific evaluation methods in the program's strategic evaluation plan on a yearly basis to assess student learning and comprehension of equitable care practices	

Developing a Metacognition Philosophy for APN Practice

Similar to developing a nursing theory-based philosophy for practice, a metacognitive philosophy can assist the APN in driving the use of metacognition as a tool for innovation. According to Lovett (2008), metacognition is a necessary skill for creativity, critical thinking, and problem solving, the three essential skills for each APN to assert into their roles and practice. As with each skill learned in nursing, metacognition takes time to master. It may take some time to gain a full understanding of the impact the skill will have on how we learn, think, and create. Being in the APN's role can produce more time constraints for metacognitive practice, yet the necessity of the skill is recognized and required for APNs to make positive impacts on patients, peers, and students. Another benefit of adopting a "reflect-in-practice" philosophy can inspire other colleagues and nurses to see a model of the process and its subsequent impact on the APN's role. Transitioning from a reflective practice to one in which the APN can reflect in practice can be positive and a means of building personal satisfaction. Using metacognition in a cyclical way leads to deliberative practice with a greater retention of new knowledge.

Creating a Reflect-in-Practice Philosophy

To commit to a new process or method of practice, we need to generate value. The same is true for learning a new skill, like metacognition. Metacognition is a conscious effort and demands a commitment to self-awareness. Even Aristotle stated the importance of reflection, believing it has a role in developing practical insight and understanding one's own imagination (Contreras et al., 2020). The philosopher John Dewey associated life experiences and education by viewing experiences as an essential part of learning, with a connection made between thoughts and actions through reflection (Contreras et al., 2020). Nursing education has used reflection as a learning tool since the 1980s (Bulman et al., 2012). Despite its long-standing history and endorsements, metacognition is often undervalued for its effects on nurses and APN practice.

The pandemic created problems that by no means can be viewed in linear fashion with one-size-fits-all solutions. Rather, the issue facing health care now and in the future will require more insight and creativity to make constructive impacts on all people to support health and wellness. Creating value to metacognition, or a reflect-in-practice philosophy, asks the APN to take the necessary steps to understand the process and commit to integrating to one's own practice. As APNs gain further knowledge of nursing theory as a tool with the use of metacognition, synergy in their practice and interactions within their roles is created. The proposed use of theory aligned with metacognition will lead to a new sense of awareness for the APN to mitigate health care challenges while adding innovative solutions along the way.

> *"We are all on a journey of self-discovery—the quality of that journey depends on who, if anyone, is navigating."*
> *—Socrates (Fine & Burnyeat, 1992)*

To create value, steps to building a reflect-in practice philosophy are offered. The APN uses these steps to gain personal insight into individual values, beliefs, and professional ethical standards. As part of this process, the APN will explore patient, student, colleague and other interprofessional views to gather a holistic perspective with the full intent to discover more about self and what we value as a person and as a nurse/APN. The steps will assist the nurse/APN to determine the value in committing to a reflect-in-practice philosophy while learning about what is important to their unique journey as a nursing professional.

TABLE 5.6 Steps to Building a Reflect-in-Practice Philosophy Focused on Using Metacognition

Steps	Description	Link to APN roles
1. Commit to reflect in practice.	Develop an awareness and allow for curiosity to provide value in exploring all scientific, theoretical, and philosophical inquiries related to your APN role.	*APN clinician*: Seek continued education in a specialty field with an emphasis on patient care and outcomes. *APN leader*: Seek competency-based education in leadership and management while exploring new models of leadership. *APN educator*: Seek new models and theories for education and pedagogy to enhance student learning and teaching practices.
2. Formulate key questions.	Build a list of questions pertaining to your role in health care directed toward a justification to your role.	*APN clinician*: Construct questions for clinical practice directed at the mission of the institution and align each with your personal values. *APN leader*: Construct questions aligned with models of leadership you wish to employ based on your values and beliefs. *APN educator*: Construct questions on direction of curriculum to explore and integrate theoretical underpinnings and nursing values.

TABLE 5.6 Steps to Building a Reflect-in-Practice Philosophy Focused on Using Metacognition (*Continued*)

Steps	Description	Link to APN roles
3. Study human nature.	Explore your experiences in nursing while seeking to understand humanity from multiple perspectives to ensure a holistic approach.	*APN clinician*: Evaluate interactions with patients and pause to reflect on the outcomes to answer why a certain outcome occurred. *APN leader*: Evaluate interactions with administrators and other leaders to consider actions and reactions in specific situations. *APN educator*: Evaluate interactions with student and fellow educators (clinical and academic) to understand needs in the learning environment.
4. Discern criteria for truth.	Establish a set of truths regarding health care and its mission to serve people while relating to your specific role.	*APN clinician, leader, and educator*: Ask discerning questions to fully understand the mission and vision of the health care setting you are practicing in to determine alignment with your values and professional ethical standards.
5. Reconcile beliefs with criteria.	Resolve your beliefs/values to the setting-established criteria to ensure intellectual integrity and pursuit of progress.	*APN clinician, leader, and educator*: If criteria do not align with your values, reconcile the difference and adjust accordingly.
6. Conduct a self-assessment.	Quantify your knowledge, skills, abilities, strengths, weaknesses, and interests and develop a vision of who you want to be within your APN role.	*APN clinician, leader, and educator*: Create one or more professional APN goals and align your current strengths and weaknesses to determine gaps in knowledge.

(*Continued*)

TABLE 5.6 Steps to Building a Reflect-in-Practice Philosophy Focused on Using Metacognition (*Continued*)

Steps	Description	Link to APN roles
7. Seek peer review.	Seek out interdisciplinary and interprofessional colleagues to discuss major points of view to test your philosophy for consistency and intellectual integrity.	*APN clinician*: Speak with other APN clinicians and providers to ascertain others' values and efforts in providing care to patients. *APN leader*: Speak with other nurse leaders, managers, and professional administrators to ascertain values and ideas on upholding current policies and in creating new policies to strengthen health care delivery systems. *APN educator*: Speak with other educators (clinical and academic) to ascertain values and methods of instruction to strengthen core pedagogical beliefs and educational models.
8. Evaluate.	Create feedback mechanisms to evaluate ongoing changes in values, beliefs, and organizational goals.	*APN clinician, leader, and educator*: Implementing a consistent evaluation method ensures your commitment to reflection in practice is ever-evolving and offers the prospect for continued professional improvement over time.

Positive Response for the APN to Apply to Multiple Practice Settings

Whether in the clinical, organizational, or academic settings, a reflect-in-practice philosophy will lead the APN to employ successful metacognition. APNs will be better at monitoring, comprehending, and problem solving. The building of a reflect-in-practice philosophy will engage the APN to use intentional questioning and model techniques, leading to self-regulated, lifelong learning. As the APN learns to use metacognition, the skill becomes inherent and intentional without the need of prompting. The process will lead into professional fulfillment by gaining a sense of accomplishment and "making an impact." The goal is to facilitate action in the promotion of quality care.

The APN clinician can impact clinical settings by engaging in a more purposeful approach to patient care needs and by interacting in a positive manner with colleagues. A practice built on a philosophy (or more than one) creates value, which in return drives action(s). The APN leader can impact the organizational setting by creating synergy between administration, staff, and patients focused on safeguarding a proactive, equitable, and value-driven care approach. The APN educator can impact future nurses and APNs by engaging in assessment of curricula and educational goals to serve students in a way that prepares them holistically to care for humans across the life span.

> Confucius, a Chinese philosopher, once observed three ways to acquire the necessary wisdom you need for life:
>
> "By three methods we may learn wisdom: First, by reflection, which is noblest; Second, by imitation, which is easiest; and third by experience, which is the bitterest."

CHAPTER 6

Metacognition Process

Key Terms

Burnout (nurse): An emotional response to work, characterized by the following dimensions: emotional exhaustion (EE), or the feeling of inability to provide a service to others; depersonalization (D), reflected as animosity or cynical behavior toward others; and low feelings of personal accomplishment (PA), evidenced by decreased self-confidence, intolerance to frustration, and impaired job performance (Membrive-Jiménez et al., 2022).

Constructivism: Learning takes place when new information is built into and added onto an individual's current structure of knowledge, understanding, and skills (Mambrol, 2020).

Emotional intelligence (EI): The ability to manage one's emotions and the emotions of others while promoting the well-being of nurses, which subsequently impacts patients and families (Raghu Bir, 2018).

Mindfulness: An awareness that arises through paying attention, on purpose, in the present moment, nonjudgmentally (Kabat-Zinn, 2018).

Self-assessment: A reflective process in which students use criteria to evaluate their performance and determine how to improve (Siegesmund, 2017).

Self-awareness: Aims at developing a contextual and relational awareness of one's emotional states and outlooks, meaningful life patterns, actions, beliefs, and preconceived ideas influencing daily personal and professional interactions (Rasheed et al., 2019).

Introduction

As nursing is often described as a discipline in transition, nurses and APNs are accustomed to the fluctuating work environment, which increases patient acuity with a need for comprehensive education and wide-ranging leadership actions. Nursing on the surface understands learning is ongoing; however, tools and strategies to promote higher intellectual engagement leading to innovation are often under-reported or overlooked without offering a supportive framework. The questions remains: How do we know what we know and what we don't, and how do we apply new knowledge to practice? The answer can be found in *metacognition*.

Metacognition offers personal insight while linking past, present and future knowledge. The process calls for nurses and APNs to have active ownership over learning before, during, and after experiences. In part, a constructivist viewpoint is adopted. Under constructivist principles, learning occurs when knowledge is both constructed and deconstructed. In other words, learning is most effective when knowledge is constructed with meaning. The "deconstructed" knowledge is accomplished in the ability to use self-assessment. Self-assessment requires students to self-regulate learning based on individual ability to utilize metacognition. As nursing theorist Patricia Benner (2012) describes the expert nurse as having a sense of fluidity enabling the nurse/APN to move in and out of practice specialties (and practice levels), so does metacognition. Metacognition offers a flexible

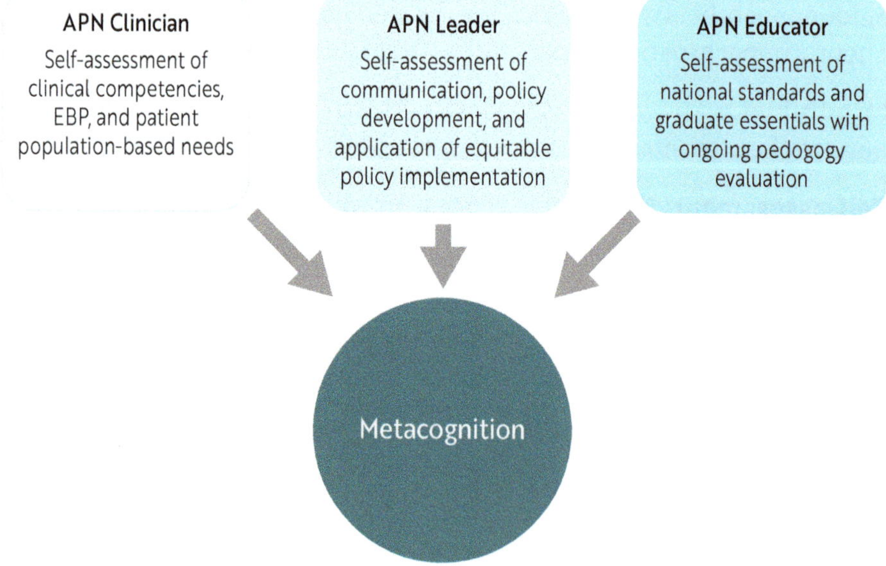

FIGURE 6.1 Relationship between self-assessment and metacognition.

process to assist the nurse/APN to reach the level of an expert nurse who can internalize metacognition to manage, anticipate, and create opportunities for quality, safe nursing practice.

As APNs embrace metacognition as a process to enhance professional practice, tools and strategies will need to be in place to support them. A common goal in the metacognition process is to transfer and/or implement discoveries from reflection to practice. The call for metacognition asks the APN to raise self-awareness above the subject matter to include gaps in knowledge and bias responsiveness. Becoming active in monitoring self-efficacy through understanding strengths and weaknesses creates a strategy for the APN to engage in a high level of competence in both intellectual and social skills. Challenging the APN to adopt a cognitively active philosophy promotes synergy in each respective role.

Metacognition has distinct attributes to be understood by the student, nurse, and APN. Metacognition's core is self-awareness. As metacognition calls for a reflective capacity, self-awareness underpins this principle and can facilitate successful implementation of the metacognitive process. Self-awareness allows the nurse/APN to focus on critical issues to begin the process of regulating what is known and what needs to be understood to adapt practice to a higher level of skill and level of quality care. Stemming from self-awareness are independent, control, and proactive attributes. Independent, as an attribute, relates to the individualized nature of metacognition. Reflection is unique to the individual's experiences and knowledge. Control places the power of the process in the individual, compelling the APN toward self-regulated learning. The proactive attribute builds a sense of action in a positive manner. The APN actively seeks new and reinforced knowledge to influence their roles and performance in practice. Distinguishing metacognition explicitly for the APN can empower a sense of professional satisfaction and contribution to the art and science of nursing.

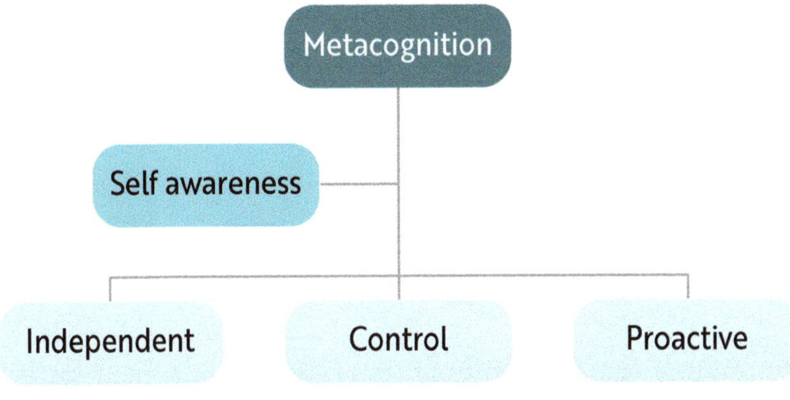

FIGURE 6.2 Metacognition attributes.

The chapter will address the following learning objectives:

1. Illustrate tools for the APN to apply to an individualized metacognition process.
2. Appraise strengths and weaknesses as an essential element of the metacognition process.
3. Examine the metacognition process through cognitive action employing skilled strategies.

Metacognition Tools

Tools or resources are essential components to any learning experience. As students, we have used various learning strategies to assist in taking preferred knowledge to long-term (usable) memory. Days have passed since memorization was a method of learning. Considering the complexities of the health care environment with many moving parts, the APN is subject to "thinking on our feet." This reflexive concept of APN practice assumes each decision is made with certainty and based on evidence. By adding a reflect-in-practice philosophy, the APN can optimize their thinking (clinical reasoning) to enrich practice, navigate evidence, and consider innovative responses.

Mindfulness/Clearing the Mind

Amid an often-rushed health care environment, APNs feel pressure to complete responsibilities and fulfill obligations in caring for patients, leading change in health care settings, and ensuring a sound educational experience for students. The profession of nursing is demanding both mentally and physically and is unpredictable. In addition to the challenges faced in practice, emotions can wax and wane, creating a symphony of exhaustion and frustration. To manage these (un)certainties, APNs can equip themselves with tools, such as mindfulness, to use metacognition as a supportive means of providing the best care, leadership, and education.

Reflective Pause

How many times can you remember walking into a supply room and needing to recall what were you going in there for?

Mindfulness enables a sense of presence, or an in-the-moment feeling. This sense of awareness provides a clearing of the mind from distractions and puts the APN on a path to think without reaction. Mindfulness allows the mind to do its job with greater effectiveness, whether in a quiet meditation or during day-to-day activities. Being mindful promotes a sense of presence and interaction with your thoughts and the environment around you without judgment. Thinking without judgment is aligned with acceptance of the process. Establishing a personal goal to enhance professional skills, knowledge and attitude can promote an objective sense of personal feelings and what we know and do not know to create a pathway to learning.

Mindful Meditation: A Tool for Nursing Survival

In these post-pandemic times, managing work–life stressors through mindfulness, as a tool for successful use of metacognition, is needed more than ever to support APNs. Due to the demands of the APN in a highly flux environment, auto pilot becomes evident in practice, with our minds traveling at the speed of light, either anticipating future events or ruminating over something that has happened. The American Nurses Association's (2016) health risk appraisal report found that 82% of nurses believe they're at a significant level of risk for illness due to workplace stress. Nurses and APNs experience physical and emotional exhaustion, which can lead to depersonalization and detachment from their roles as care providers, leaders, and educators. Some have aligned these feelings to nurse burnout. Traditionally, nurse burnout is perceived as an individual issue, yet the effects on the health care system are daunting and supported by studies indicating a relationship to less patient safety, decreased quality of care, poor patient satisfaction, and a decrease in nurse commitment and productivity (Jun et al., 2021). Nurse burnout has been evaluated using Maslach's Burnout Inventory, a scientific tool focused on emotional exhaustion, a cynicism subscale, and a single-item measure of self-defined burnout (Knox et al., 2018). Calming the mind and gaining focus on one's nursing career is both healthy and productive for the individual APN and the organization.

Maslach's Burnout Inventory: Application for the Advanced Practice Nurse

To enhance your understanding of the application of Maslach's Burnout Inventory, check out the following article exploring strategies for advanced practice nurses to reduce work stress:

Klein, C. J., Dalstrom, M., Weinzimmer, L. G., Cooling, M., Pierce, L. M., & Lizer, S. (2020). Strategies of advanced practice providers to reduce stress at work. *AAOHN Journal*, 68(9), 432–442. https://doi.org/10.1177/2165079920924060

Practicing mindful meditation can provide significant physiological and psychological benefits for the APN. Reduction of stress, anxiety, and burnout and enhanced resilience have been claimed as outcomes of mindful meditation (Van Der Riet et al., 2018). The practice of mindfulness can help APNs achieve more satisfactory outcomes the next time an overwhelming situation occurs. Through the process of actively engaging in mindful meditation, the APN learns that stress is manageable, with the potential to result in a more effective, efficient outcome. In a study by Penque (2019), mindful mediation resulted in statistically significant results in the three primary outcomes associated with Maslach's Burnout Inventory, personal accomplishment, emotional exhaustion, and depersonalization, providing validity to mindful meditation for nursing survival.

TABLE 6.1 Principles of Mindful Mediation for the APN

Principle	Rationale
Acknowledge bias.	Focus on a nonjudgmental approach by finding awareness of your perceptions, beliefs, and values.
Acknowledge perseverance.	Perseverance and commitment to patience in the process provides the opportunity to live in the moment.
Acknowledge learning.	Value learning as ongoing process that is ever-changing, allowing your mind to be open and embrace personal/experiential knowing.
Acknowledge intuition.	Allow yourself to trust yourself while letting your ideals guide you with a commitment to open listening.
Acknowledge uniqueness.	Practice an understanding that you are enough and there is no need to be different; rather, each moment of mindful meditation leads to enhancing who you are.
Acknowledge acceptance.	Recognize interprofessional and interdisciplinary disagreements and embrace situational facts.

Mindful meditation directs the APN to care for self as an extension of Watson's self-care theory. Even though psychological wellness may need a multiprong approach, such as employer-sponsored initiatives, mindful meditation places the APN in control of individual practice and leadership. Through the action of mindfulness, we give ourselves space for thought, for breath, and between ourselves and (gut) reactions. Despite mindfulness being a natural process, it may take time and dedication to practice regularly and with intention.

Mindful meditation can be a survival tool and a learning strategy that impacts the APN's role in a positive and satisfying way. APNs understand the challenges they face in their unique roles and often become robotic in their practice while focused on caring for others at all costs. Avoiding negative reactions to overgiving of self can be quite beneficial to the APN and provide the opportunity to grow personally and professionally.

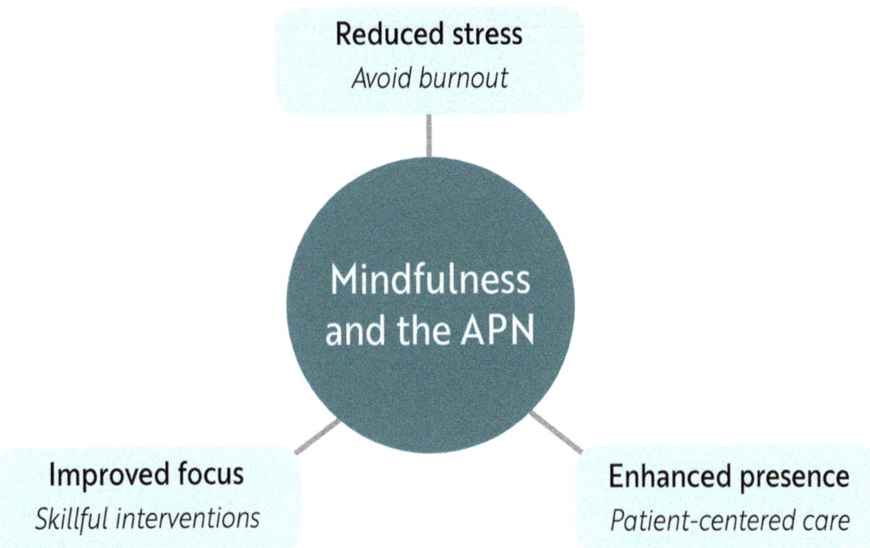

FIGURE 6.3 Benefits of practicing mindfulness for the APN.

TABLE 6.2 Tips for Practicing Mindful Mediation for the APN

Tips of Mindful Meditation	Considerations for the APN
Create a daily routine/commit.	Use meditation as a tool on a regular basis and begin by selecting time that is uninterrupted.
Expand mindfulness as both an activity of perception and observation.	Reflect on times when you felt at ease, and think of how you felt. Try using meditation and breathing exercises to accept this time for self-reflection.
Expect anxious feelings.	A quiet moment may bring on emotions such as restlessness and irritation. Recognize the emotions as expected and use a nonjudgmental approach to embrace new thought processes.
Travel with mindfulness.	No matter the activity you are engaged in, mindfulness can be active in your thought processes, cultivating positive responses.
Accept each mindful moment for what it is.	Avoid judgment of each mindful moment as either good or bad. There is no bad mindful meditation, only growth and learning.

Mindful Meditation: A Tool for Nursing Innovation

Calming the mind can benefit the APN by generating opportunities for creative thought. Nurses and APNs alike have been called to be change agents and lead health care delivery improvements grounded in a value-based approach. Clearing the mind, using deliberate thought processes, and staying in the moment can enhance the APN's creativity in solving issues and concerns within each unique APN role. It is worth asking if mindfulness can assist APNs to connect more to issues within nursing practice, leadership, and education.

To make a comparison to nursing, characteristics often described of mindfulness mirror the characteristics associated with transformative leadership, which has been widely recognized and utilized in nursing practice: emotional intelligence (EI), clarity, focus, energy, empathy, and patience. Health care organizations encourage the use of transformative leadership in nursing as a positive outcome resulting in higher patient satisfaction. The parallel between transformative nursing and mindfulness manifests through effective communication and enhanced (positive) attitudes, creating a healthier work environment. According to James MacGregor Burns (2010), the author of *Leadership*, transformative leadership occurs when two or more persons engage with others in such a way that the leader and followers raise one another to high levels of motivation and morality. The description by Burns (2010) supports APN practice, whereas mindfulness becomes a tool to engage wholly into transformational leadership, creating a pathway to innovative practice.

Transformative Leadership and Impacts of COVID-19

For more information on transformative leadership and the impact of COVID-19, please review the article provided:

Fowler, K. R., & Robbins, L. K. (2022). The impact of COVID-19 on nurse leadership characteristics. *Worldviews on Evidence-Based Nursing, 19*(4), 306–315. https://doi.org/10.1111/wvn.12597

For so many nurses, a proud nursing moment may have come from being creative or innovative in responding to a patient's need, a staff concern, or even a teaching moment. These moments of satisfying creativity may be fleeting compared to being consistent as nurses are overworked and stressed. To gain a wider perspective, mindfulness, or present-centered attention, has been surging in many industries, such as Google, Aetna, Mayo Clinic, and the U.S. Army, to promote and improve workplace functioning (Jha et al., 2015). Research in such disciplines as psychology, neuroscience, and medicine provides a wealth of evidence that mindfulness affects attention, cognition, emotions, behavior, and physiology in positive ways (Jha et al., 2015).

Researching Mindfulness and Impact on Creativity

For more information on research of mindfulness and its impact on workplace creativity, please review the article provided:

Byrne, E. K., & Thatchenkery, T. (2019). Cultivating creative workplaces through mindfulness. *Journal of Organizational Change Management, 32*(1), 15–31. https://doi.org/10.1108/jocm-10-2017-0387

While creativity cannot be forced or produce ideas steadily, APNs can apply a systematic approach to individual practice to find and engage in the right conditions to generate innovation. APNs should be encouraged and become deliberate in training the self to participate in a multitude of experiences within their unique specialty practice. This intentional engagement in experience(s) is known as being omnivorous. Omnivorous encourages the APN to seek a breadth of experiences that nurture the APN to be more open and flexible about practice experiences. The APN generates an intentional focus on immediate, present, and future experiences, often reframing the perception of risk or unfamiliarity from fear or frustration to opportunities for growth. One method to dissuade the fear and frustration is to employ a simple technique known as STOP, a type of meditation in which the person raises a sense of awareness while sensing in the moment without interpretation and judgment (Graff-Radford, 2022). The STOP meditation technique assists the APN to be present in the moment. Often rushed environments, such as health care, can be overwhelming and fast-paced, leading the nurse and APN to juggle the thinking process without the opportunity for synthesis in decision-making.

S Stop what you are doing and pause.

T Take some deep breaths.

O Observe the experience in the moment just as it is.

P Proceed by checking what is needed right now.

FIGURE 6.4 STOP: A mindfulness technique.

Mindfulness can not only inspire the APN in practice but also through organizational goals. Mindfulness under a business framework can explore concepts associated with team learning and building (collaboration), supportive leadership, and adoption of employee innovation initiatives. As health care strives to improve workplace conditions and create a culture that supports sustainable methods to stay current, mindfulness can prove to be an organizational effort to support employee innovation. Engagement is a critical concept between organization and employee. According to Jain et al. (2018), a working environment with jobs that are designed to enable psychological safety, learning opportunities, voice and supportive leadership is susceptible to proper health, safety, and wellness management and thus in support of sustainable economic performance and innovation. As mindfulness continues to gain momentum in research to impact organizational sustainability, the act of mindfulness can serve as a tool for innovation, creating a pathway for nursing's voice to be instrumental in integrating moral, adaptive, and technically sound practice approaches to patient care, leadership, and education.

Assessing Strengths and Weaknesses

Being authentic is synonymous with being a nurse. Many attributes of nursing are linked to nursing's ethical standards, such as beneficence, justice, and fidelity. Authenticity is a measure of knowing oneself through identification of individual strengths and weaknesses. The process of discovering one's strengths and weaknesses can be daunting and intimidating but is an essential task for the APN to practice holistically. The overarching goal for discovering one's strengths and weaknesses is self-awareness.

Self-awareness is an essential nursing competency (Rasheed et al., 2020). Self-awareness is described by Rasheed et al. (2019) as a contextual and relational awareness of one's emotional states and outlooks, meaningful life patterns, actions, beliefs, and preconceived ideas influencing daily personal and professional interactions. Becoming self-aware is a requirement for personal and professional growth, allowing the APN to recognize their potential offerings to their unique practice specialties while maintaining control of their professional performance. There are multiple instruments available for the APN to employ to discover strengths and weaknesses, and for the purpose of this text and the alignment to mindfulness and innovation, a strengths, weaknesses, opportunities, and threats (SWOT) analysis will be explored.

TABLE 6.3 APN Benefits of Self-Awareness

Benefits	APN Clinician	APN Leader	APN Educator
Cultural Competence	Discovery of exposure to different patient demographics served in specialty areas	Discovery of staff and management interactions with recognition of bias to policy development	Discovery of curriculum designed to teach cultural care across the life span
Decision-Making	Discovery of added critical thinking skills integrating EBP to treatment modalities	Discovery of implementation of policies with adherence to ethical standards and organizational goals	Discovery of student assessment in recognition of clinical reasoning and judgment
Therapeutic Relationships	Discovery of therapeutic relationships between provider and patient as well as disciplinary and interdisciplinary colleagues	Discovery of therapeutic staff and managerial relationships to create a safe and supportive workplace environment	Discovery of student and patient engagement to foster skills associated with therapeutic relationships
Holistic Practice	Discovery of bias impacting care intended to address body, mind, and spirit of all patients	Discovery of bias impacting staff and managerial relationships	Discovery of bias in curriculum development and student assessment tools

SWOT

The SWOT analysis tool was originally created in the 1960s as a business/brainstorming strategy to analyze similarities and differences between an organization and its competition (Teoli & An, 2019). A SWOT analysis provides the APN with awareness of critical issues with a focus on both internal and external factors, ultimately influencing the APN's actions (practice). According to Teoli and An (2019), strengths and opportunities are facilitators that assist the APN to achieve set goals, whereas threats and weaknesses are barriers in achieving set goals. The application of SWOT analysis is broad but can be an individualized tool for the APN. Commonly used questions can be applied to address each category of the SWOT analysis to provide the APN with a strategic professional plan to apply tools such as mindfulness and nursing theory to achieve full-scope, integrative, holistic, and innovative practice.

TABLE 6.4 Common Questions for APNs to Employ a SWOT Analysis

SWOT	APN Clinician	APN Leader	APN Educator
Strengths (Internal Facilitator)	What do I do well to serve the population of patients in my practice setting?	What service(s) do I bring to my department/setting that has enabled better performance of my staff?	What educational experience(s) do I bring to enhance courses taught and learning opportunities for students?
Weaknesses (Internal Barrier)	What do patients and colleagues see as limitations to my full scope of practice?	What do my staff and peers see as limitations to my authority to oversee organizational goals?	What do my colleagues and students/nurses see as limitations to my ability to serve as a role model aligned to concepts taught?
Opportunities (External Facilitators)	Are there (new or existing) opportunities I can seek to enhance my clinical practice?	Are there (new or existing) opportunities I can seek to enhance my administrative practice?	Are there (new or existing) opportunities I can seek to enhance my educational practice?
Threats (External Barriers)	What existing or potential issues could impact my ability to provide holistic care?	What existing or potential issues could impact my ability to oversee and lead organizational initiatives?	What existing or potential issues could impact my ability to implement, revise, and assess educational objectives?

From the responses of the SWOT analysis, the APN can plan to improve, address, and seek professional growth and in real time adjust practice. Self-awareness is a product of the SWOT process, allowing the APN to embrace areas of improvement while addressing areas of proficiency and expertise. In many aspects, the SWOT analysis can be used as an assessment technique aligned with Benner's novice to expert theory. The acknowledgement of the results of a SWOT analysis can assist the APN in navigating current practice and future professional endeavors or accomplishments. As the APN engages in tools like the SWOT analysis, it is helpful to highlight nursing philosophies and review criteria associated with the goals and vision for individual professional development.

The SWOT analysis can be viewed from multiple viewpoints, which can further tailor the tool for the APN. Additional viewpoints can include recipient, community, and learning and growth perspectives. Under the recipient perspective, the APN can seek insights from the viewpoint of the patient, staff, or student. The APN invites questions that pursue an understanding of the experience of interactions between self and those who receive care, guidance, and education from the APN. From the community perspective, the APN seeks insights regarding the impact their roles have on the community they serve, from geographical to demographic attributes. The community perspective engages the APN to seek a broader understanding of the population they serve. And, from the learning and growth perspective, the APN seeks insights into personal and professional ways to reach goals through identification of resources.

When to Use a SWOT Analysis as Part of the Metacognition Process

Metacognition is proposed as a tool to be used on a continuous basis, whereas the SWOT analysis can be done as a method to evaluate the APN's overall progress toward goals and current performance. Often, a SWOT analysis is implemented prior to a substantial change, such as transitioning to a new position or advancing scope of practice. However, as an extension of metacognition, a SWOT analysis can be done as an ongoing assessment with the purpose of discovering new initiatives for the APN to explore within their unique role as clinician, leader, or educator. The timing of the SWOT analysis will be dependent on the APN and their career trajectory. As a result, the SWOT analysis develops into an innate method of self-reflection directing the APN toward goal development and adjustment.

Implementation of the SWOT analysis assumes the APN sees value in its application. The APN student can begin the use of the SWOT analysis during the beginning, middle, or end of their respective programs. A comparison should be measured to understand the ongoing benefits a SWOT analysis can provide the APN. In addition, the new APN in practice should reassess every 3 months for the 1st year to discern the value of the tool in gauging and directing their practice roles. Once the APN has completed using the tool, a timeframe can be established based on the APNs goals. The most essential element to the use of the SWOT is to compare previous analyses to identify patterns and gaps in resources to assist the APN in meeting goals.

How to Use a SWOT Analysis as Part of the Metacognition Process

A common application of the SWOT analysis is to use a visual aid with a four-square diagram depicting each area. Broad or specific questions can be applied based on the perspective the APN is assessing (recipient, community, or learning and growth).

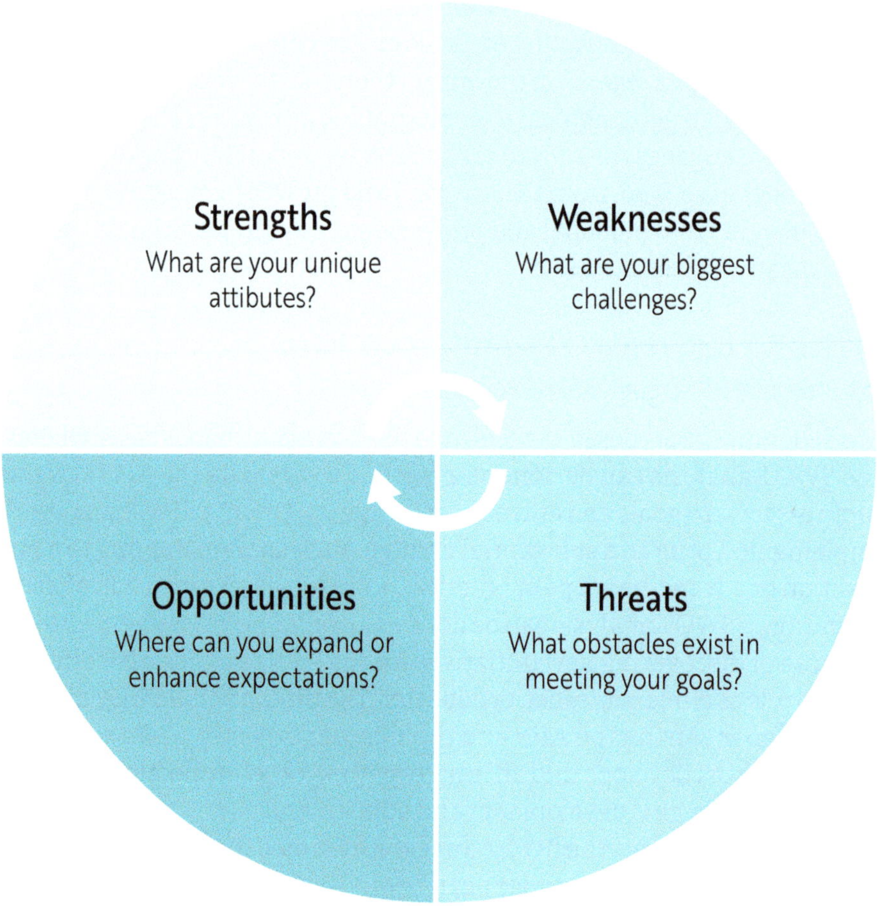

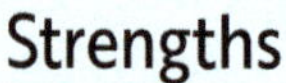

FIGURE 6.5 Visual example of a SWOT analysis.

Once the visual aid is selected, the APN should gather information. Using objective information will best serve the APN in evaluating without bias. The key to gathering information is to first select the right questions to ask in each domain. The selection of questions will be based on the perspective and the role of the APN. Once the questions have been selected, the APN will need to employ metacognition (mindful meditation) prior to answering each question. Allowing one's mind to calm and contemplate answering each question without pressure or prejudice can enhance the process and result in a positive impact on the APN's career and current role.

APN Metacognition Skill Strategies

Metacognition skills specific to the APN can prove to be a valuable as well as supportive tool for an organization. The gains from metacognition are

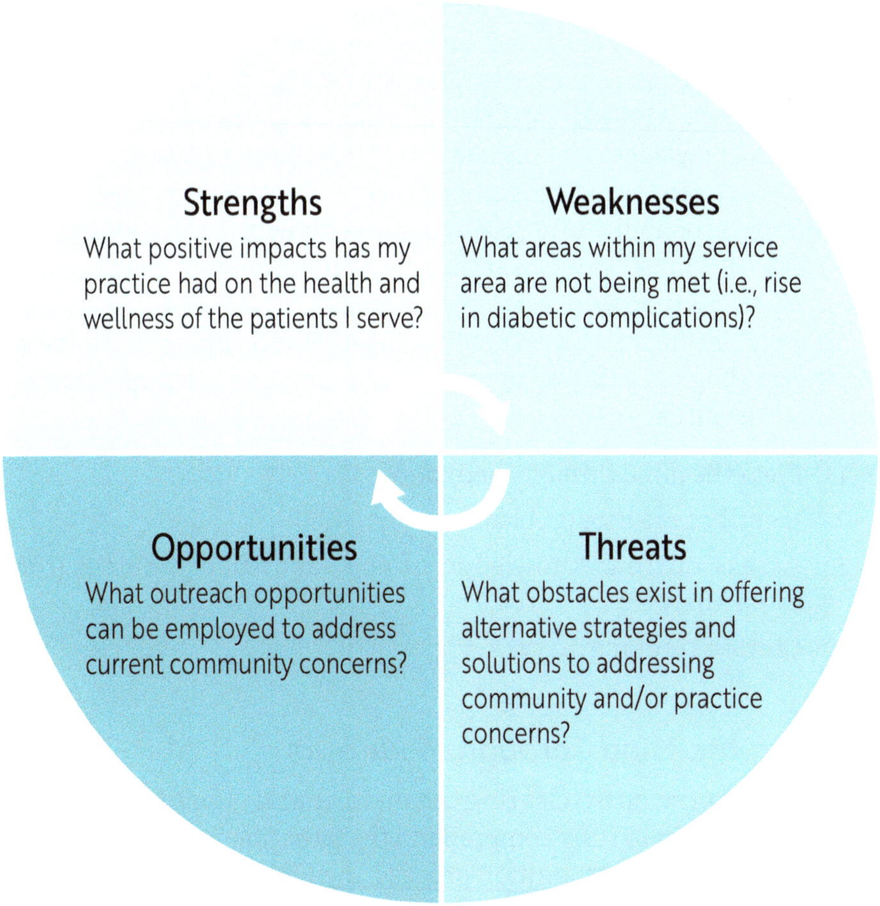

FIGURE 6.6 Example SWOT analysis for the APN clinician/community perspective.

vast and should be explored on both personal and organizational levels. Not only will the participant of metacognition enhance problem-solving and reasoning skills but will also actively self-regulate lifelong learning and professional growth. These skills are developed as a result of intentional questioning (SWOT analysis) and metacognition (mindfulness). To successfully engage in a metacognitive process, three phases of metacognition need to be understood: metacognitive knowledge, metacognitive monitoring, and metacognitive control (Dunlosky & Thiede, 1998).

Before applying metacognitive-specific skill strategies for the APN, metacognitive knowledge should be recognized as the information gathered during the time of investigating an idea, issue, or concern. For the APN clinician, this can equate to standards of care or EBP. The APN leader acknowledges leadership strategies, existing and desired, to improve continuity in the workplace setting. The APN educator recognizes various pedagogies or educational theories to structure curriculum and learning strategies for a variety of student needs. Metacognitive monitoring is the ability to assess cognitive activity (Dunlosky & Thiede, 1998). In the monitoring phase, the APN evaluates the information gathered and if there are any gaps in knowledge. Seeking additional information (data or resources) creates synergy in the metacognition process. The final phase, metacognitive control, is the ability to regulate cognitive activity (Dunlosky & Thiede, 1998). The APN must be aware of the time commitment of metacognition and apply ample time to invest into its process.

To apply the metacognition process, the APN will engage in the following steps to begin a pathway of professional ongoing learning and steps towards innovation:

1. Clear the mind through meditation.
2. Identify a practice problem.
3. Assess current knowledge of the identified problem (root-cause analysis).
4. Create a thinking diary.

Clearing the Mind Through Meditation

As discussed previously, clearing the mind enables the APN to be present in the moment to fully comprehend the situation without judgment. In this step of the metacognition process, the APN focuses on a particular idea, issue, or concern in the attempt to train awareness and achieve a mental and emotional calm state. Through awareness, the doorway to introspection and self-reflection is opened. As the APN calms the mind, the analytical drive begins to proceed and peel back the layers of the idea, issue, or concern. Through this awareness, a higher order of thinking occurs with a conduit toward theorizing without emotional attachment. By allowing a clearing of the mind, the APN creates space for learning and a level of intelligence unattached to subjectivity. The mind is given the opportunity to think without judgment and reactivity, creating cognitive space for synthesizing innovation.

Identifying a Practice Problem

As the APN clears the mind, a topic is selected to begin the process of metacognition. Depending on the specialty role, the APN can select practice problems (issues) to focus on conceiving solutions. Using metacognition, the APN has more freedom in selecting practice problems. For many APNs, specific problems can become lost in the rush of day-to-day practice. Limited time to explore problems can lead to frustration and a loss of empowerment for the APN. Employing a metacognition process gives back a sense of empowerment and control to the APN. Whether the problem is clinical, administrative, or education based, the APN has a set pathway to use a 30,000-foot view and a thought stream driven to find, create, and evaluate solutions.

Assessing Current Knowledge of the Identified Problem

As the APN focuses on a specific problem to address, a critical step is to discover and appraise existing knowledge about the problem (issue). In this strategic phase of metacognition, the APN will need to be open to receiving objective and subjective data about the problem. Many times, a problem may not be identified until a subjective (negative) inference is observed, often leading to seeking a deeper understanding of the problem. An effective, and nonjudgmental way to assess current knowledge is to use root-cause analysis (RCA).

RCA is a collective term that describes a wide range of approaches, tools, and techniques used to uncover causes of problems. Multiple RCA tools can be utilized, such as a fishbone diagram to map the potential causes of a problem. The goal of RCA is to identify what happened, why it happened, contributing factors, and how to prevent it from happening again. RCA methods are like metacognition as each uses a reflective approach. RCA seeks answers to solving problems while reducing risk or harm. The use of RCA tools can vary and be selected based on the APNs preference and alignment with the problem being investigated.

TABLE 6.5 RCA Tools to Explore for Each APN Role

RCA Tool	APN Clinician	APN Leader	APN Educator
Fishbone diagram https://www.cms.gov/medicare/provider-enrollment-and-certification/qapi/downloads/fishbonerevised.pdf	✓	✓	✓
Pareto chart https://www.ihi.org/resources/Pages/Tools/ParetoDiagram.aspx		✓	
Five whys analysis https://www.cms.gov/medicare/provider-enrollment-and-certification/qapi/downloads/fivewhys.pdf	✓		✓

Creating a Thinking Diary

As the APN goes through each phase of metacognition, a thinking diary can benefit the process by having a designated space to arrange ideas, thoughts, resources, and impressions of the effort(s) dedicated to metacognition. Whether this space be written, typed, or recorded, the thinking diary offers the APN an opportunity to assess thinking or cognitive activities. Here, the APN uses all three phases of metacognition: metacognitive knowledge, monitoring, and control.

As metacognition is a fluid process that occurs over time, the thinking diary can be evidence of the possibility of change. As the field of psychology has deduced, cognitive activity affects behavior. Many times, as APNs we employ models to change behavior in others to seek improved health, workflow, and learning. The thinking diary can be a strategy to support APNs in doing the same in a constructive and positive approach. Cognitive techniques, such as a thinking diary, can encourage the APN to challenge their thinking and understanding to new, different ways of thinking, opening the door to innovation.

Figure Credit

PART III

Aligning Theory to Five Prevailing Post-Pandemic Health Care Challenges

Even as the pandemic created obstacles, hardships, and changes in the very fabric of cultures and societal norms, we would be remiss to not look at this time in history as an opportunity for growth through transition. Health care change is seen in how we prepare providers, use technology to serve as a primary care service, expand disease-prevention awareness, and supply chain forecast, to name a few. APNs hold a distinctive position within health care and the profession to be change managers and adopters of best practices to ensure safe, quality, and accessible care management and education.

In Part III, an exploration of five prevailing post-pandemic health care and educational challenges will be outlined based on the impact to the system at large and within the framework of the nursing metaparadigm: health, person, nurse, and environment. The nursing metaparadigm represents the core of what it is we do as nurses. It provides central themes and unifying concepts that form the basis of nursing. As each of the five challenges are discussed through the nursing metaparadigm, nursing theories and models will be identified as resources, or tools for the APN clinician, leader, and educator to use in their diverse roles.

The five prevailing post-pandemic health care/educational challenges explored are as follows:

- remote care/education
- health care costs/education costs
- poor patient/student outcomes

- health care/educational disparities
- ethical challenges
    - nurse's safety
    - patient/student safety
    - role and moral distress
    - resource allocation
    - APN clinician–patient relationship
    - APN leader–staff relationship
    - APN educator–student relationship

Each of the five health care and educational challenges are marked as having substantial impacts to the APN's responsibilities and patient, staff, and student experiences. The APN clinician, leader, and educator will have different encounters with each of these challenges yet face significant effects on their unique roles. By enhancing the APN's insight of these health care and educational challenges in the post-pandemic era, nursing theories can be valued as pragmatic and not abstract contexts within the academic arena.

CHAPTER 7

Aligning Theory to Remote Patient Care and Education

Key Terms

Authenticity: The quality of being what is professed in origin and as being genuine (Oxford English Dictionary Online, 1989).

Health: A state of complete physical, mental, and social well-being and not merely the absence of disease or infirmity (WHO, n.d.a.).

Interpersonal relationships: The interaction between two or more people who communicate and transfer values and energy from their roles in society (King, 2007).

Telehealth: A larger umbrella term encompassing other remote health-related services, such as administration, continuing medical education, and/or provider training (Shaver, 2022).

Wellness: An active process through which people become aware of, and make choices toward, a more successful existence (Cross, 2020).

Introduction

Bridging care from tertiary care to the home and offering virtual educational technologies has been increasing since the pandemic. Multiple studies prior to the pandemic concluded patient satisfaction with virtual health visits being preferred over face-to-face visits and a consensus of ease of use, low-cost, improved communication, and elimination of travel time (Kruse et al., 2017). Despite the overall positive perceptions of virtual health care platforms, telehealth services were underused (Shaver, 2022). A major reported drawback of telehealth from both patient and provider perspectives was the potential for "impersonal" encounters and rising concerns over personal data security. These concerns created a reason for telehealth to be stagnant in adoption across the health care spectrum. Medicare and Medicaid services prior to the pandemic had limitations to the application of telehealth as evidence in the following regulations:

- Only certain licensed providers could implement telehealth services.
- Only patients with a preexisting condition could use telehealth services.
- Only designated sites, such as rural areas could use telehealth services.
- Only Medicare coinsurance and deductibles apply to telehealth visits.
- Only preapproved technology platforms can be used for telehealth visits. (CMS.gov, 2020)

These restrictions (and many more) slowed the progression of telehealth as a usable, effective, and dynamic addition to health care delivery. During this stagnation of telehealth adoption, complex, chronic diseases skyrocketed, creating a looming need for enhanced communication and connectivity between patient and provider and resulting in potential loss in translation or missed opportunities for follow-up care. Then COVID-19 hit and the telehealth model for remote health care became a lifeline for patients, providers, leaders, educators, and students.

Shelter-in-place and many other recommendations to distance from one another surged the use (or need) of telehealth to maintain connectedness to providers for care management while making virtual learning platforms a necessity to continue to offer specialized education. Prior policies and restrictions of telehealth services were rapidly relaxed, and a collective effort between insurances (state and private) and Congress paved the way for telehealth to be energized as an effective mode to serve patients across multiple specialties. In addition to virtual health care delivery, APN leaders and educators adopted technology platforms to create synergy for communicating and educating while adhering to guidelines to protect groups from the transmission of the virus.

Growth of Telehealth During COVID-19

A national study of 36 million working-age individuals with private insurance claims data showed that telemedicine encounters increased 766% in the first 3 months of the pandemic, from 0.3% of all interactions in March to June 2019 to 23.6% of all interactions in the same period (Weiner et al., 2021).

Even from the expansion of telehealth and remote communication and educational platforms, the question remains of how telehealth will continue to adapt to the changing health care and educational landscapes. Informational technology continues to grow the advances in health monitoring and virtual learning environments with a benefit of reducing barriers such as time, distance, and mobility. Many concerns will remain, and this is when APNs can make an impact with the aid of tools like nursing theory and metacognition to guide their efforts. There are multiple nursing theories and models that can be viewed to assist the APN, but for the purpose of broadening the usability of nursing theories, a variety of theories will be explored under each of the nursing metaparadigm domain to address each of the five prevailing post-pandemic health care challenges. This chapter will explore the following learning objectives in relation to remote health and education challenges:

1. Explore the nursing metaparadigm through the challenges set forth post-pandemic with remote care and education.
2. Align selected nursing theories and models to each domain of the nursing metaparadigm: health, person, nurse, and environment.
3. Analyze the role of APN clinician, leader, and educator to meet the challenge of remote health care and education through the lens of innovation.

Nursing Metaparadigm: Health

Defining health has transformed since the onset of the pandemic. People have become hypervigilant of what it means to be healthy and strive for wellness as an outcome. Health is considered a multidimensional concept, including the holistic view. Health as one of the four domains of the nursing metaparadigm refers to a dynamic process focused on the synthesis of wellness and illness and is viewed based on an individual's perception across the life span. Health is a context and is relative, whereas wellness is the lived experience of feeling cared for and illness is the lived experience resulting in a loss of function. The degree of health is premised on mutual interactive processes between people and their environment. As the pandemic ensued, health became a tangible outcome for many who may have overlooked the risk of illness. The dramatic change of remote health care and education became a necessity, causing an adoption of newer technologies. Expectations have also changed since the pandemic in that patients anticipate a faster response from providers. Students in educational settings also look for ways of reaching educators in a more streamlined, technological approach with minimal wait time. Societal experiences with technology have expanded in a way that makes convenience and immediacy an expectation rather than just a benefit of technology. As remote platforms continue to intersect both health care and educational settings, APNs have a critical role in addressing these expectations with ease of implementation and responsive solutions as challenges evolve.

For many experts in the health care arena, telehealth holds a strong promise to improve preventative care initiatives and be considered a disease-prevention tool for health care providers. Not only is the reach of telehealth broader, but it can provide enhanced workflow for providers, with streamlined access to patient health information. The concept of convenience may be debated in telehealth applications; however, the use of technology to influence patients does have added approachability while offering alternative methods for follow-up care, time for patient questions, and provider explanations of care interventions and preventative recommendations.

In consideration of chronic care management, telehealth can reach patients directly regarding certain behaviors, such as weight management. Patients can implement and promote their own health. Telehealth, or remote care, and its associated technology places a sense of autonomy in the hands of the patient. Being placed in a waiting room, filling out endless papers, and finding the transportation to various health care visits taxes many patients and creates a negative response in that the patient may not follow up with care or adhere to prescribed care interventions. The remote health visit creates an environment for the patient to be prepared to spend uninterrupted time with their care provider, creating a synergy effect between the provider and the patient.

In the educational environment, remote learning has opened many doors for learning and accessibility of various educational options. Despite the need to prepare students for the expectations within remote learning environments, the online platform enhances autonomy, often expanding students' experience to reflect on learning. The online platform creates prospects for students to develop strong communication skills and collaborate with others while learning from peer experiences. One critical aspect of online learning has been debated, and this relates to mental health. The potential for isolation does exist and should be recognized as a potential risk. As health is an ongoing concern for students, advanced practice educators must consider the way the platform is developed to ensure student interactions, active learning strategies, and ongoing review of remote learning pedagogies.

Health is a precious, individualized state for all people. APNs from clinical to leadership and education should be aware of the need to assess health in all interactions, whether it is patient, staff, colleagues, or students. Since the pandemic, health has become a major concern for people worldwide.

The palpable need to be healthy has increased and will continue, requiring APNs to be cognizant of the ways we reach people and provide care, direction, and education. Health, as a concept, is a process where one's life experiences influences a person's capability to strive and maintain a path towards health and wellness. Through this concept, nursing reviews health as operational to promote the benefits of a healthy lifestyle. Health has been and is a building block for nursing theory. Nursing theory can provide guidance in this area by addressing how we can teach others to conserve and reduce risk(s).

Health: Levine's Conservation Model for Nursing

In analyzing health as a concept and the role of the APN, it may go without saying a nurse/APN would explore Pender's health promotion model or Watson's self-care theory. Both would be excellent options; however, a broader view of nursing theory is offered to assist the APN student to explore the potential practical use of nursing theory to each APN specialty role (clinician, leader, and educator). Myra Levine's conservation model is an example of this broadening perspective of using theory to guide advanced practice.

The conservation model at its core is designed to improve a person's physical, spiritual, and emotional well-being by addressing four key domains of conservation: energy, structural integrity, personal integrity, and social integrity. The alignment to holism is evident. Defining each of the domains is an important step for the APN:

- Conservation of energy refers to balancing energy input and output to avoid excessive fatigue, including adequate rest, nutrition, and exercise (Levine, 1967).
- Conservation of structural integrity refers to maintaining or restoring the body's structure, preventing physical breakdown, and promoting healing (Levine, 1967).
- Conservation of personal integrity recognizes the individual as one who strives for recognition, respect, self-awareness, selfhood, and self-determination (Levine, 1967).
- Conservation of social integrity exists when a patient is recognized as someone who resides within a family, a community, a religious group, an ethnic group, a political system, and a nation (Levine, 1967).

Levine's model assumes everyone is an active participant in interactions with the environment, constantly seeking information from it. As for the concept of health, Levine (1967) describes health as the pattern of adaptive change of the whole being. To fully understand the assumptions of Levine's model, defining adaptation and conservation is necessary:

- *Adaptation* is the process of change and integration of the organism in which the individual retains integrity or wholeness (Levine, 1967).
- *Conservation* includes joining and is the product of adaptation, including nursing intervention and patient participation, to maintain a safe balance (Levine, 1967).

Additional Articles on Levine's Conservation Model

Read more about the application of Levine's conservation model in nursing practice:

- Monaro, S., Pinkova, J., Ko, N., Stromsmoe, N., & Gullick, J. (2021). Chronic wound care delivery in wound clinics, community nursing and residential aged care settings: A qualitative analysis using Levine's conservation model. *Journal of Clinical Nursing, 30*(9–10), 1295–1311. https://doi.org/10.1111/jocn.15674
- Kirca, N., & Özcan, Ş. (2022). The effects of nursing care based on Levine's conservation model on fatigue, depression, perceived social support, and sleep quality in infertile women: A randomized controlled trial. *International Journal of Nursing Knowledge, 34*(4), 284–296. https://doi.org/10.1111/2047-3095.12402

In addressing the use of telehealth and remote education, Levine's conservation model can speak to the APN clinician, leader, educator, patient, employee, and student in a myriad of ways, all supporting each role in achieving health as a positive outcome. The transition to remote delivery is ongoing and will continue to unfold throughout the health care spectrum. Health, as nursing domain, includes the concept of accessibility. Remote care and educational platforms offer a wider range of accessible options. Adaptation, as defined by Levine, will provide direction for the APN to address issues associated with remote care and education. For the APN, adaptation will enhance practice skills while answering the call for flexibility in highly flux environments, such as primary or tertiary care and educational settings. As Levine suggests, the environment in which a patient or student is in will include internal and external aspects, all of which will influence one another. A person's environment will be complex, and it is through the assumptions of adaptation and conservation that APN clinicians, leaders, and educators can assist in creating environments that support and promote health. Whether the environment is health care or educational settings, remote access will be a growing platform calling for APNs to be skilled and knowledgeable and have positive attitudes about its applications.

TABLE 7.1 Achieving Health Through Remote Delivery: Usability of Levine's Conservation Model for APN Clinicians, Leaders, and Educators

Conservation Domains	APN Clinician	APN Leader	APN Educator
Conservation of Energy	To practice with insight of patient's needs by using deliberate interventions to balance activities and the patient's available energy and resources. To use remote health services to reduce burden to patient in seeking health care.	To offer leadership and managerial skills equipped with providing support, resources, and attention to staff needs while considering workloads (demands) of staff. Use of remote IT applications to engage in full stakeholder input.	To design and implement effective learning strategies that reduce time while increasing comprehension, adding to student's knowledge base. To use remote learning platforms to decrease cost and burden to students seeking advanced educational opportunities.
Conservation of Structural Integrity	To use clinical judgment in choosing care interventions with minimal side (adverse) effects. To use remote health care to effectively assess in a timely manner without delay in care or interventions.	To use a leadership framework that offers tools to inspire without impacting staff resiliency. To use remote delivery of meetings to ensure timely responses to policy changes or needs.	To include active learning strategies that engage students to learn actively without burdening students with additional cost and resources. To use remote learning platforms or meetings to expedite discussion among faculty/administrators and students to preserve student integrity related to academic progression.

(Continued)

TABLE 7.1 Achieving Health Through Remote Delivery: Usability of Levine's Conservation Model for APN Clinicians, Leaders, and Educators (*Continued*)

Conservation Domains	APN Clinician	APN Leader	APN Educator
Conservation of Personal Integrity	To include patient in care decisions and actions toward health. To use remote health services to include the patient and promote patient autonomy in seeking health care.	To use a transformative approach to include staff and stakeholders in important unit/setting decisions. To use remote platforms to increase staff input and feedback.	To engage in a student-centered approach to teaching and evaluation. To use a remote platform to decrease anxiety and increase student feedback in academic progression needs.
Conservation of Social Integrity	To include social support per patient's network in care planning. To use remote care applications to include family/social networks approved by the patient to enhance patient inclusion in care and address specific care needs/resources.	To include staff and all related employees impacted by unit/setting oversight as a method of support and feedback. To use remote platforms and applications to promote unity among staff by supporting their voice in critical unit/setting decision-making.	To seek faculty colleague and student feedback in curriculum design and implementation. To use remote platforms to increase student and faculty responses without bias or intimidation.

Person: Watson's Theory of Caring and Travelbee's Human-to-Human Relationship Model

Person, under the context of the nursing metaparadigm, includes the one on the receiving end of care, and for the purposes of the APN educator, the student, and the APN leader, staff/colleagues. There are multiple facets to the person domain, which include spirituality, culture, social network, and individual SDOH, such as socioeconomic status. The person can be extended to include the community (specific populations), or even an institution. To discuss person as a domain of the nursing metaparadigm, it is essential to consider the whole person: mind, body, and spirit.

To care for a person requires honoring their wishes, customs, and beliefs. If nursing excludes one facet of a person, it can diminish the healing process, or the continuum of wellness. In the context of applying theory to the person domain regarding remote care and education, it is critical for the APN to be authentic and present to not only demonstrate dignity of the person but also be active in the relationship process. Remote health care and education do and will have ongoing challenges to ensure a sense of connectedness required to care and teach. Authenticity can be used to define or prepare a foundation for providing remote care and learning platforms. Due to the nature of a person and their unique needs, a genuine display of presence is a necessity to effectively support remote care and education. Jean Watson's theory of caring and Joyce Travelbee's human-to-human relationship model will serve as guides for the APN to address remote care and education through the person domain.

Watson's theory of caring is premised on the transpersonal relationships established between people. For the APN, it is an assumption to create a practice that follows principles of caring across the spectrum of human nature without bias or judgment. Watson (1985) suggests caring is seen through a unitary worldview promoting the use of all ways of knowing, engaging in teaching, and learning experiences, creating a caring and healing environment, valuing humanity, and embracing unknowns. To further analyze the assumptions laid forth by Watson, the APN can align the theory's assumptions to create, manage, and evaluate remote platforms. Watson's theory of caring has served as a framework for many nursing initiatives to inspire professional practice models and research to promote exceptional human-to-human caring practices. Through the application of Watson's theory, the APN can find meaning in day-to-day practice, resulting in resiliency for the APN and authentic experiences for patients, staff, colleagues, and students.

As the pandemic quickly instilled a sense of isolation across the globe, caring became an imminent need for many. With the fast adoption of remote health care services and educational learning environments, a sense of community began to form. Ongoing use of remote platforms cannot be unnoticed as a mainstay and requires acknowledgement of the need to create connection and authentic experiences for the providers, patients, educators, and students. The understanding and use of Watson's theory of caring can provide a guide to instill a true connection between persons. Watson's theory guides the APN to offer authentic presence and intentionality to optimize an experience for the patient, student, staff, and colleagues while in a remote environment (platform).

Joyce Travelbee's human-to-human relationship model focuses on concepts related to existentialism in that humans are constantly facing choices and potential conflicts while being accountable. Due to the model's notion of human choice, mental health becomes a central point of exploration. Choices can be complicated and need guidance. While working within a remote environment, choices can become overwhelming without a life preserver. The APN can recognize this phenomenon and address the need

TABLE 7.2 Applying Watson's Theory of Caring in Remote Environments for the APN Clinician, Leader, and Educator

Watson's 10 Curative Factors	APN Clinician	APN Leader	APN Educator
Embrace	To practice with acknowledgement of altruistic values and kindness to all persons	To lead with altruistic values and kindness to staff, colleagues, and peers	To teach through altruistic values and kindness to students and colleagues
Inspire	To practice with a sense of hope and honor for others' uniqueness	To lead with a sense of hope and honor for all persons engaged in policy and practice development	To teach with hope and honor all students' paths to learning
Trust	To practice by nurture and promote patient personal growth	To lead by nurturing staff and colleagues while offering opportunities for growth and development	To teach through a sense of nurture with the intent to enhance the learning process for all students and colleagues
Nurture	To practice with the pure intent to help others	To lead by trusting others to follow and demonstrate understanding	To teach within a trusting environment
Forgive	To practice by being present for positive and negative circumstances	To lead through both positive and negative circumstances while staying open to others' perceptions	To teach while recognizing others' experiences as a process of learning
Deepen	To engage in lifelong learning by seeking out best practices	To engage in ongoing evaluation of processes to ensure safe, current, and flexible pathways	To teach with a sense of duty to understand, apply, and evaluate various pedagogies for learning
Balance	To practice by seeking to understand individual needs and readiness to change	To lead by recognizing the need for change while embracing the courage to make change	To teach based on the understanding of each person's unique learning style
Cocreate	To practice with a deep respect for human dignity by acknowledging one's preferences or opinions	To lead by creating a healing environment in which all can experience mutual respect	To teach based on the premise of mutual respect between educator and student

TABLE 7.2 Applying Watson's Theory of Caring in Remote Environments for the APN Clinician, Leader, and Educator (*Continued*)

Watson's 10 Curative Factors	APN Clinician	APN Leader	APN Educator
Minister	To practice by striving to meet each person's individual physical, emotional, and spiritual needs	To lead by engaging in a holistic approach regarding all areas of management	To teach with the appreciation of each student's holistic needs, supporting cognitive growth through experience(s)
Open	To practice with an appreciation and recognition of the unknown, creating an open and welcoming environment for the patient	To lead with gratitude and a sense of knowing change and challenges will occur	To teach with an open mind, allowing for student cognitive development and sharing of the process

for human-to-human connections as surmised in Travelbee's model.

> *"We must continually question the value of our achievement, continue learning, and actively seek to improve our ability ... to gain increased understanding of our human condition."*
>
> *—Travelbee (1963, p. 72)*

In reviewing Travelbee's model, one may see an alignment to clinical specialty areas, such as palliative care. As this would be a natural association, the assumptions laid forth in Travelbee's model can be forged in new and innovative ways based on the underpinnings of connection and authentic encounters. A common theme in many nursing theories and models is interpersonal relationships. The necessity of the APN creating a mutually beneficial relationship cannot be understated. As remote technologies advance and become integrated in more aspects of everyday life, the awareness of a loss of connection to others must be identified and evaluated. According to Travelbee (1971), the nurse is responsible for educating and providing strategies to assist the patient in avoiding or alleviating the distress of unmet needs. As the APN seeks to understand a person's needs, they too explore through self-reflection to better relate to patients, students, staff, and colleagues on a human-to human level. A major concept in Travelbee's model is to fully understand what a human being is. "A human being is a unique irreplaceable individual—a one-time being in the world, like yet unlike any person who ever lived or ever will live" (Travelbee, 1971, p. 26). The APN seeks to know the person on an individual level, connecting in a way that creates the desired interpersonal relationship. The understanding that humans are ever evolving can provide a prompt to APNs to know their efforts to assist, guide, and educate are beneficial and necessary.

As health care systems strive for person-centered care and educational institutions strive for student-centered learning, Travelbee's model supports the movement to make these important human-to-human connections. Travelbee (1971) included five phases that envelop the human-to-human relationship:

1. the initial meeting or encounter
2. the visibility of personal and emerging identities
3. empathy
4. sympathy
5. establishing mutual understanding and rapport

Each of the phases requires skilled communication. It is through communication that the APN can create an interpersonal relationship. Skilled communication lies in the APN's understanding of a person's human actions and how they are influenced by earlier life experiences. As a major assumption of Travelbee's model is placed on suffering; it leaves the concept open to interpretation based on unique human experiences. As the APN evaluates the role technology is playing in health care and education, the need for interpersonal relationships remains and should be evaluated within remote platforms.

Nursing: Peplau's Theory of Interpersonal Relations and King's Theory of Goal Attainment

Nursing theory has historically provided a definition of who we are and what we do. Nursing can be defined in many ways based on a multitude of specialty practices. In reference to the metaparadigm and to offer a broad description, nursing is a science with a body of knowledge that has arrived through theory development, research, and logical examinations. Many refer to nursing as both an art and a science focused on holistic care guided by ethical principles and values, which include autonomy and responsibility. Nurses are called to use this body of knowledge in creative ways to apply therapeutic interventions. Caring is a central focus of nursing practice, and it requires a commitment to authentic interactions exhibiting empathy and mutual respect for all persons across the life span.

Nursing utilizes clinical judgment to facilitate translation of nursing knowledge, skills, and technologies to provide care, leadership, and learning opportunities. The role of the APN is highly complex and asks the APN to engage as a learner, clinician, leader, and educator to responsibly use

TABLE 7.3 Applying Travelbee's Five Phases of Building an Interpersonal Relationship in Remote Environments for the APN Clinician, Leader, and Educator

Travelbee's Five Phases of Building an Interpersonal Relationship	APN Clinician	APN Leader	APN Educator
The Initial Meeting or Encounter	To see the person and not only an expectation of the person and their needs	To see the staff and colleagues without biased perceptions of their needs	To see the student with a clear view of their learning needs
The Visibility of Personal and Emerging Identities	To embrace the person as dynamic with unveiling personal attributes and needs	To embrace the staff and colleagues as evolving and adapting to change(s)	To embrace the student as a lifelong learner with expanding knowledge
Empathy	To understand the person's position from their unique perception	To understand the staff and colleagues from their point of view and position within the unit	To understand the student from individual life experiences
Sympathy	To show compassion through all person interactions	To show compassion in all aspects of management and leadership endeavors	To show compassion to student needs during the learning process
Establishing Mutual Understanding and Rapport	To share with the person experience(s) in reaching health and wellness	To share with staff and colleagues' accomplishments and recognize the need for change(s)	To share student achievements and recognize challenges to learning

diagnostic, technologic, supportive, and therapeutic care to safely influence and improve health among all people. The goal of nursing is to be humanistic and provide deliberate and systematic, goal-oriented interactions with the intent to empower others. Two nursing theories, Peplau's theory of interpersonal relations and King's theory of goal attainment explore the APN's commitment to provide professional nursing interactions while working within remote environments.

Peplau's theory of interpersonal relations focuses on the relationship constructed between provider and recipient. A specific assumption of Peplau's theory is to use every interaction as an opportunity for empowerment. As remote environments continue to develop and offer alternative means to access care and education, APNs can support the person by engaging in a relationship that encourages and inspires self-efficacy. There is an underlying need for a partnership between the person and the APN, and Peplau

(1997) furthered this assumption by offering three stages for the APN (nurse) to identify and engage in a therapeutic relationship:

1. orientation phase
2. working phase
3. termination phase

At each phase the APN meets different needs of the person and fulfills various roles, such as resource person, teacher, surrogate, and counselor (Peterson, 2013).

TABLE 7.4 APN Roles in the Three Phases of Peplau's Theory of Interpersonal Relations

Peplau's Three Phases for Building Interpersonal Relations	APN Roles	APN Skills Needed
Orientation Phase	Resource person Surrogate Counselor	Active listener Unbiased Person centered Diplomatic Mindful Technical expertise
Working Phase	Leader Teacher	Creative (innovate) Independent (autonomous) Approachable
Termination Phase	Communicator	Articulate Assertive Persuasive Supportive

Amid the remote (virtual) settings of health care and education, a core requirement of APNs is to care and communicate proficiently and with empathy. The nature of health care and education is transitioning to an on-demand model. The essence of nursing must be emphasized and integrated in all platforms of person-to-person interactions. Following Peplau's phases can guide the APN to enter interpersonal relationships while upholding caring interactions, even as different providers and educators interact with persons at different time intervals. The phases offer consistency and systematic frameworks for building and maintaining interpersonal connections.

Imogene King's theory of goal attainment centers around the nurse–person relationship in that each person brings perceptions of self, their role and personal growth, and development levels (King, 1971). King's theory strives to identify behaviors to decide on interventions to achieve mutually agreed-on goals. The role of the nurse according to King is to promote, maintain, and restore health. The interaction(s) between person and APN requires a transaction that is perceived as accurate by both parties. In further evaluation of the concept transaction, the impetus is placed on the person as an active participant in goal setting and health attainment (Schub, 2016).

According to King (1971), nursing is a process of action, reaction, and interaction with a sharing of information, knowledge, and perceptions of a given situation. Based on this shared information, specific goals and concerns can be addressed to achieve a mutually agreed-on goal(s). A major assumption of King's theory is that nursing should be focused on human beings interacting with their environment to lead to an improved state of health and the ability to function in social roles. Under the category of assessing remote settings, which requires interactions between APNs and patients, students, staff, and colleagues, the remote environment has the potential to influence outcomes and requires the APN to be cognizant of potential challenges. To address potential challenges, APNs can look to King's focal themes of communication and interaction. The APN develops skills to holistically interact while utilizing appropriate and consistent communication techniques, which are adapted to meet the person on their level of understanding.

> *"Nursing is a process of action, reaction, and interaction whereby nurse and client share information about their perception in the nursing situation."*
>
> *—King (1971, p. 11)*

Included in King's theory is the concept of synergy. Synergy enhances interpersonal relationships in a way that supports goal setting and goal achievement. King describes three synergistic systems to assist in reaching goals listed as follows:

- personal system
- interpersonal system
- social system

Each system can be viewed as having its own supporting concepts. APNs in clinical, leadership, and educational settings can utilize these systems when addressing remote setting platforms.

Environment: Hall's Care, Cure, Core Theory

The environment encompasses the physical, emotional, and social surroundings of the person. The environment is highly influential on a person's health and well-being as well as the success of achieving individual goals. The environment is to be assessed as fluid and changeable to sustain adaptation as an essential factor of achieving goals. To understand the environment in the context of the nursing metaparadigm, the person and the environment

TABLE 7.5 Applying King's Three Phases of Goal Attainment in Remote Environments for the APN Clinician, Leader, and Educator

King's Three Phases of Goal Attainment	APN Clinician	APN Leader	APN Educator
Personal System	To evaluate and appreciate the person as a whole being	To evaluate and appreciate the staff and colleagues as whole beings with individual contributions to the whole system	To evaluate and appreciate the student as a whole learner with multiple influences from personal experiences
Interpersonal System	To acknowledge the interaction between provider and person as essential to achieve goals	To acknowledge the interactions among staff, colleagues, and leaders as a collaborative partnership to achieve goals	To acknowledge educator and student interactions as joint relationship to achieve learning
Social System	To utilize social networks to enhance the decision-making process while governing behavior toward goal achievement	To utilize the organization as a support system to assist staff, colleagues, and leaders achieve system-based goals	To utilize the educational institution as a structured support network to assist students in achieving higher education goals

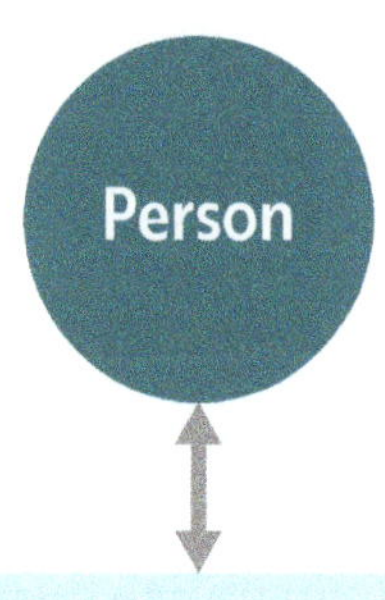

FIGURE 7.1 Example environment factors: Internal and external.

are seen as contiguous. The APN is called on to view the environment as an extension of the person and their unique daily truths. The influence from both internal and external environments is strong and highly evidenced as being either oppressive or supportive in one's journey.

Lydia Hall's care, cure, core theory focuses on a major assumption that the person is the motivation and energy needed to achieve goals with three major concepts: individual, health, and society and the environment. Hall's vision was placed into three spheres, care, cure, and core. Each of these spheres change based on the person's needs and dynamic state of health. The core sphere encompasses the body, or the person at the receiving end. The care sphere encompasses the APN. The cure sphere is the interventions used to attend to the needs of the person. Each sphere is independent yet connected to achieve goals. In remote settings, Hall's theory can offer the APN a new vision for assessing the needs of the person while maintaining a consistent relationship in a remote setting calling for full participation by both parties, the APN and the patient, student, staff, and/or colleague.

> *"To look at and listen to self is often too difficult without the help of a significant figure (nurturer) who has learned how to hold up a mirror and sounding board to invite the behaver to look and listen to himself. If he accepts the invitation, he will explore the concerns in his acts. As he listens to his exploration through the reflection of the nurse, he may uncover in sequence his difficulties, the problem area, his problem, and eventually the threat which is dictating his out-of-control behavior."*
>
> *—Hall (1965, p. 2)*

As each sphere is interrelated, the APN can address the needs of the person while acknowledging how it can change based on the growth and development of the person. The APN can use their understanding of the environment in alignment with care, cure, core to plan appropriate communication, assessment, and interventions.

CHAPTER 8

Aligning Theory to High Health Care Costs

Key Terms

Adaptation: Occurs when people respond positively to environmental changes (Roy, 2011).

Bureaucracy: Complex systems with political, legal, economic, and technological dimensions (Ray, 1989).

Bureaucratic: An integrated system in organizations to maintain the quality of health care (Lusiyana et al., 2019).

Differential caring: A dynamic social process that emerges as a result of the various values, beliefs, and behaviors expressed about the meaning of caring (Ray, 1989).

Gross Domestic Product (GDP): The value of the goods and services produced in the United States (U.S. Bureau of Economic Analysis [BEA], n.d.).

Health care consumer: An individual who uses the services of a health care provider, including patients receiving medical care or treatment (IGI Global, n.d.).

Health care spending: Number of services delivered per person × number of people to whom services are delivered × average cost of each service (Grover, 2022).

Probabilistic thinking: A belief in a conditional world in which the expectation of continual certainty and predictability is abandoned (Mishel, 1988).

Transition: "A passage from one life phase, condition, or status to another" (Schumacher & Meleis, 1994, p. 239).

Uncertainty: The inability to determine the meaning of illness-related events, occurring when the decision-maker is unable to assign definite value to objects or events or is unable to predict outcomes accurately (Mishel, 1988).

Introduction

Prior to the pandemic, in 2016, the United States spent nearly twice as much as 10 high-income countries on medical care and performed poorer on many population health outcomes (Papanicolas et al., 2018). Even though health care utilization remained the same, the main drivers for increasing costs were related to prices of goods and labor, such as pharmaceuticals and administrative costs (Papanicolas et al., 2018). Many attest the U.S. health care system is unsustainable, with a large percentage of spending related to rising prices. The APN is an essential member of the U.S. health care system and invaluable when it comes to voicing a nursing perspective in assessing data to inform policy decisions that affect the bottom line for the health care consumer.

Health care spending can be viewed as a simple algorithm: Dollars charged for health care services used. Exploring the causes of increased health care spending needs to be viewed in a multiprong approach. Some causes are related to changing demographics, such as a large percentage of Americans getting older, and other causes may be fiscally related, such as price. Closely examining the causes of increased prices for health care can guide the APN in their distinctive roles to have the greatest impact on services provided. By understanding causes such as the expansion of technology into health information, evaluation of waste from insurance and provider payment systems, and current assessment of aggregate data of the types of illnesses seeking care, APNs can positively impact those they serve whether it is through care, management, or education.

The nursing profession strives to ensure people have access, affordability, and equity in care and education. As discussed previously, value-based care is a major initiative to drive health care payment based on incentives for outcomes and value. APNs can have a significant role in transitioning to new payment models with a focus on a higher degree of interoperability and widening access for people in the post-pandemic era. Despite some initiatives to implement VBC, continued declining patient, system, and educational outcomes need to be acknowledged. Outcomes such as lower life expectancy, higher infant mortality rates, and higher prevalence of chronic diseases continue to plague U.S. health care systems (Bush, 2018). A sequelae of negative impacts occur, including the following:

- People without health insurance may not seek preventative care and develop a more costly, serious medical disorder that could have been prevented.
- When employers spend more on health care, the costs of their products and services increase.

- Medical bills that are not covered by health insurance can cause bankruptcy.
- Unpaid bills result in increases in insurance premiums and taxes (Schreck, 2020).

APNs can evaluate policy through the lens of the health care consumer and recognize environmental impacts on health outcomes. It goes without saying how necessary assessing SDOH is on influencing outcomes for the person seeking care (or avoiding seeking care due to cost and limited access). As a direct line from a person's health to access to care interventions may improve their overall well-being, APNs become a lifeline, or a conduit between good versus poor health outcomes. Whether the APN functions as a clinician, leader, or educator, engagement in current policymaking while understanding the impact to patients, staff, colleagues, and students ensures health care utilization is effective and efficient, with less barriers to access.

This chapter will explore the following learning objectives in relation to increasing health care costs:

1. Explore the nursing metaparadigm through the challenges set forth post-pandemic with rising health care costs and negative impacts to health- and wellness-related outcomes.
2. Align selected nursing theories and models to each domain of the nursing metaparadigm: health, person, nurse, and environment.
3. Analyze the role of APN clinician, leader, and educator to meet the challenge of rising health care costs and negative impacts to patient outcomes through the lens of innovation.

Nursing Metaparadigm: Health and the Impact of Rising Health Care Costs

Health care costs have grown in the past 5 decades to numbers that often do not equate to the patient. In 1970, the cost of health care was estimated at $353 per person, and the cost in 2021 per person is over $12,000 (Cox et al., 2023). The overall impact health care cost can have on a country can be assessed by reviewing gross domestic product (GDP). Currently 18%–19% of the GDP is spent on health care in the United States (Cox et al., 2023). Billions more dollars are allocated to health care spending despite the pandemic effects, which did dissuade many from seeking medical care.

As advocates, APNs understand the financial strain health care spending can have on a person and their family. In July 2022, a joint report from

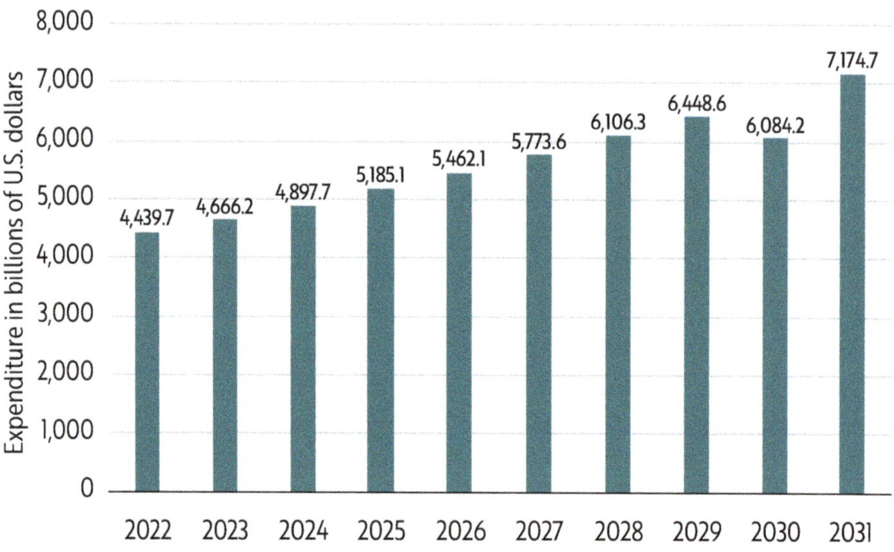

FIGURE 8.1 Growing trend of health care spending in the United States, 2022–2031.

Experian Health and PYMNTS (2022) found that a fifth of patients spent more on health care than they could afford in the previous year, causing financial distress. With current inflation rates, more and more people must decide what bills to pay versus putting food on the table. As a result, patients are postponing care, limiting prescriptions, delaying preventative screenings, and switching health care providers. Not only does the postponing of health care services impact cost through workflow disruptions, wasted clinician time, and lost revenue, it can pose health risks to the patient depending on their care needs.

According to the Kaiser Family Foundation, half of U.S. adults report having trouble affording health care costs (Lopes, Kearney et al., 2022). For the APN, analyzing aggregate data may shed light on the people in the community they serve to fully understand the impact high health care costs have on individual health. An extensive analysis is provided in Chapter 10 with aligning theory to unmask health care disparities. For a snapshot of the impact health care costs have on the uninsured, Black, and Hispanic adults, see Figure 8.2.

As discussed in previous chapters, health is defined by each person and therefore is unique in its interpretation and choice of behaviors. Inductive reasoning leads one to assume that lowering health care costs and that increasing access to care would improve a greater number of patient health outcomes; however, the commonsense thought may be too simplistic and require more critical and innovative thought to fully address the issues

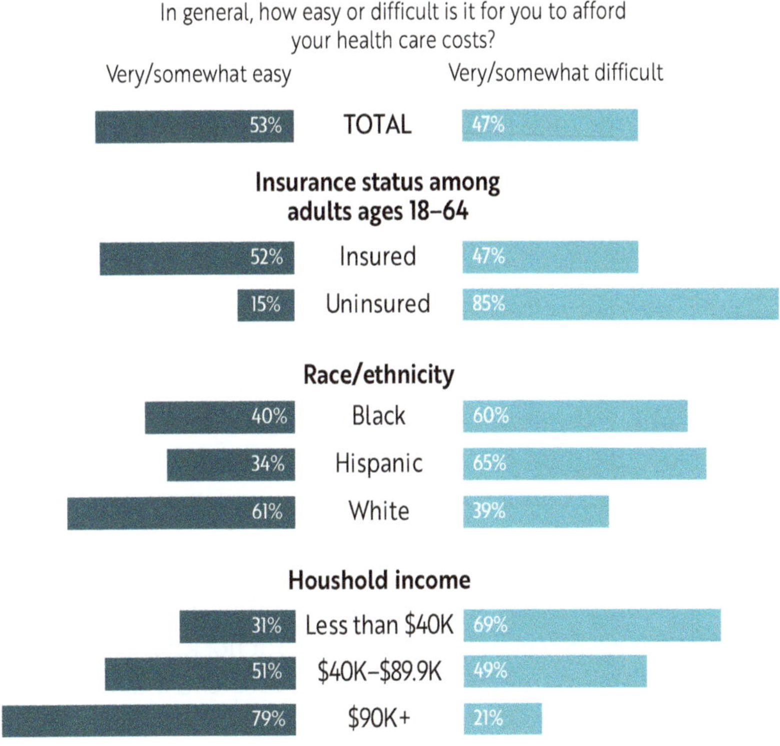

FIGURE 8.2 Uninsured, Blacks, and Hispanic U.S. adults report difficulty with health care costs.

aligned to the U.S. health care cost woes. Nursing theory can be integrated into the APN critical thinking method to assist with addressing proactive responses to population needs when seeking guidance, health goals, and means to improve living and working environments and thus influence overall health.

Health and the High Cost of Health Care: Mishel's Uncertainty in Illness Theory

Uncertainty is a concept that infiltrates and provokes every activity related to health care, from research to medical interventions at the point of care. According to the nursing theorist Merle Mishel (1988), uncertainty is the inability to determine the meaning of illness-related events, which occur when the decision-maker is unable to assign definite value to objects or events or is unable to predict outcomes accurately. Mishel's uncertainty in illness theory has been utilized in clinical specialty areas, such as oncology, to assist with explaining how the concept of uncertainty is generated and how it affects psychological adjustment. Mishel's theory will be evaluated for how uncertainty can be created because of medical debt and the inability to pay for health care, thus impacting a person's desire and actions to achieve health-related goals. Mishel's theoretical underpinnings can be applied to the APNs' roles to address uncertainty due to mounting health care costs.

To apply Mishel's theory in the context of patient uncertainty with health goals because of burdens associated with health care costs (or existing medical debts), the definition of *uncertainty* can be examined as the inability to predict outcomes accurately. Much of what health care providers witness from patients' decrease of follow-up care or postponed screenings relates to Mishel's theoretical concept of probabilistic thinking. According to Mishel (1988), probabilistic thinking is a belief in a conditional world in which the expectation of continual certainty and predictability is abandoned. The level(s) of uncertainty created due to health care cost burdens and thrusting patients into a sphere of instability subsequently causes people to not know about preventative care options and advanced avenues to treat existing diseases. A common thread with probabilistic thinking can be aligned to the lack of transparency in health care billing, or not knowing how much a treatment or visits cost until much later. This creates a misunderstanding with a diminished sense of trust in health care. No matter how engaged a health care provider is, uncertainty can ultimately influence a patient's choice to seek or not seek care.

Under the theory's major assumptions is the understanding of how uncertainty as a cognitive state represents the lack of current cognitive schemas to support interpretation (Mishel, 1988). To further deconstruct the theory, uncertainty can influence patient decision-making regarding seeking care, following up with care, and complying to prescribed health care interventions. The APN can assist the patient to identify uncertainties and support patient literacy related to health care services. Mishel's theory proposes three major themes: antecedents of uncertainty, appraisal of uncertainty, and coping with uncertainty. Each of the major themes are presented to demonstrate potential actions of each APN role to assist in overcoming the effects of high health care costs.

Mishel's theory offers four distinct dimensions of uncertainty (in illness). The four dimensions include ambiguity, complexity, deficient information, and unpredictability (Mishel, 1983). The four dimensions of uncertainty are proposed as an alignment to the impact of health on the patient, staff, and student due to the rising costs of health care.

TABLE 8.1 Applying Three Major Themes of Mishel's Uncertainty in Illness Theory to High Health Care Costs via the Roles of the APN

Mishel's Three Themes	Theme Defined	APN Clinician Action	APN Leader Action	APN Educator Action
Antecedents of Uncertainty	Anything that occurs prior to the (illness) experience that affects the patient's thinking, such as pain, prior experiences, and perception (Mishel, 1988)	Expansion of knowledge of health care resources and providing a systematic and culturally aligned method to share knowledge with patients, families, and communities	Creating an accessible pathway for staff and colleagues to obtain literature and resources with ongoing support to advance staff skills in patient and interdisciplinary communication and collaboration to reduce cost(s) directly to the patient	Researching current data on health care spending trends and effects on patient outcomes to integrate into curricula learning activities
Appraisal of Uncertainty	The process of placing a value on the uncertain situation (Mishel, 1988)	Engaging in open discussions with patients, families, and community members regarding the effects (risks) of loss of health care opportunities and resources	Sponsoring ideas to administrative leaders to decrease costs and enhance existing or create new policies that focus on VBC concepts.	Exposing students to the impacts of health care costs on patient outcomes and offering open dialogue of the impact of avoiding health care due to burdens of cost
Coping With Uncertainty	Activities that are used in dealing with the uncertainty (Mishel, 1988)	Extending resources to assist with costs of health care at the point of care and through community outreach initiatives	Empowering staff and colleagues to implement policies constructed on VBC initiatives	Teaching students to assess patient literacy on health care spending and resource options

TABLE 8.2 Mishel's Four Dimensions of Uncertainty Aligned to the Health of Patient, Staff, and Student

Mishel's Four Dimensions of Uncertainty	Patient	Staff	Student
Ambiguity	Unclear perceptions of illness	Unclear perceptions of role expectations or policy implementation	Unclear perceptions of student role and as future agents of change
Complexity	Overwhelming feelings when seeking treatment/resources	Overwhelming and inconsistent communication and understanding of policy changes impacting practice	Overwhelming complexity of curricula layout and alignment to student role
Deficient Information	Inadequate resources to meet the patient's level of understanding of illness and treatment options	Inadequate resources to support the staff in policy implementation	Inadequate resources to assist the student with understanding intricacies of health care demand versus supply (value)
Unpredictability	Instability in choosing and receiving care (options)	Instability in staff understanding why policy changes occur	Instability in student exposure and understanding of SDOH to accessibility of health resources.
Effects of Health Care Costs	Fear of seeking care due to minimal or no coverage for treatment or rising medical debt/limited income	Changing policies to meet the demands of institutional (system) needs	Lack of educational initiatives to address rising health care costs and the impact to patient outcomes with detached curricula in teaching treatment interventions to cost of care and evaluating outcomes

Guidance Through Uncertainty: A Case Study Reflection

Instructions

1. Consider your future role as an APN: clinician, leader, educator.
2. Review the provided case study.
3. Use the APN role template to guide your reflection of uncertainty.
4. Reflect on how your future APN role can address uncertainty as a major influence on outcomes: patient, staff, and student.

Case Study: Uncertainty and the APN Role

P.K. is a 45-year-old seeking care for chronic pain in his shoulder and left knee. P.K. has worked as a carpenter for 22 years and would like to continue to build his company. P.K. has a family of five, with three children under the age of 18. His wife is a schoolteacher and assists P.K. with his small company's billing. As an independent owner of a small business with eight employees, P.K. strains to offer health insurance to his employees, let alone use a health care payor for his own personal health care needs. Currently, P.K. is paying out of pocket to seek treatment from alternative providers, such as a chiropractor. He has experienced minimal relief and is now limiting job offers due to not being able to work at full capacity, creating financial and personal strain. Despite his wife's insistence to see a primary care provider, P.K. is uncertain if this will result in prolonged treatment and cost and does not want to endure additional financial strains on his family or company.

Guided Reflections		
APN Clinician	**APN Leader**	**APN Educator**
• Describe the APN clinician's reaction to this scenario. • What is a priority response for the APN clinician? • How is uncertainty going to affect P.K.'s health and life goals? • Describe three points of discussion the APN clinician would have with P.K. regarding his health and wellness journey considering uncertainty.	• Describe the APN leader's reaction to this scenario. • What is a priority response for the APN leader? • How will uncertainty affect the health care system's response when patients do not use a proactive approach to their health care choices? • Describe three points of discussion the APN leader can have with staff and colleagues in addressing similar encounters with patient uncertainty and risk of negative outcomes on the health care system.	• Describe the APN educator's reaction to this scenario. • What is a priority response for the APN educator? • How is uncertainty going to affect the patient, family, and community (company)? • Describe three points of discussion the APN educator would have with students when considering the scenario as a teaching activity to discuss the impact of uncertainty on patient outcomes and health care costs.

Person and the High Cost of Health Care: Roy's Adaptation Model of Nursing

After 3 years of the pandemic and the over 6 million COVID-19 patients, U.S. health care systems are preparing to face new challenges (American Hospital Association, n.d.). The sustained increases in health care costs are placing each system at risk for financial instability. Costs from medical supplies, rising drug prices, and workforce shortages are just the tip of the iceberg for health care systems and providers alike, not to mention the person. Persons under the domain of the nursing metaparadigm include culture, family, values, and society. The rising cost of health care is creating an overwhelming obstacle for many individuals to obtain the resources needed to guide their wellness journey. Taking care of the person is central to the APN, whether the person is a patient, family, community, staff, colleague, or student.

As inflation continues to worry many Americans along with other burdens affecting persons' desire and action to seek health care, financial instability within the U.S. health care system remains a surging concern even after the pandemic. The overall health status of Americans is declining, which can have a cyclical effect on the health care system. The increase in demand for treatments and resources can impact the need for an added workforce, enhanced technology, provider incentives, and supplementary intensive care interventions. As health declines, so are opportunities for persons to fulfill their unique roles within a community, whether managing a chronic disease, caring for family members, seeking educational prospects, or fulfilling a career passion. The APN can bring light to this bleak outlook by guiding persons to use adaptive measures to value health care as central to everyone's journey to wellness. Value in health care is measured in terms of patient outcomes achieved per dollar expended. APNs can educate patients, staff, and students to understand the costs of health care as payment not just for a procedure and item but rather based on the outcome. Outcomes are critical data to evaluate systems, providers, and care, so why not for the price of health care?

The APN can be instrumental in determining what outcome attributes should be assessed: survival, ability to function at baseline, length of care, sustainability of recovery, and educational programs. As APNs continue to practice, lead, and educate at the point of service, their contributions can enhance the measurement of outcomes and lead to a value system that places quality at the center of health care and education for the benefit of the person.

To view health care through the lens of the person, the APN needs to consider a broad perspective by including trends since the pandemic. To continue a positivist approach, the post-pandemic era is an opportunity for APNs to support and promote increased attention to individual health. More

Americans are embracing a healthier lifestyle, but this can highlight disparities. Treating the person includes the whole person, which uses a biopsychosocial approach and addresses cultural values. The rising costs of health care can prevent a true wellness journey for many, but the APN can assist people with achieving balance (adaptation) amid health challenges.

> *According to the Ipsos survey of 1,160 people in the United States, 62% of Americans believe their health is more important to them than before the pandemic. (This Is the Future of Health and Wellness, 2022)*

Roy (2011) presents the adaptation model. Roy defines *adaptation* as occurring when people respond positively to environmental changes. A major assumption of Roy's (2009) theory is the integration of human and environmental meanings, which results in adaptation. Roy adds to the theory's assumptions that people use creative abilities of awareness, enlightenment, and faith to adapt to new challenges.

Roy's theoretical assumptions can be aligned to the APN to address the need for value-based health care that is directed at equity in accessibility and knowledge of health care choice(s). By integrating Roy's four adaptive modes to the APN role, the APN can be instrumental in developing innovative paths to reach individuals and guide their options for choice, supporting adaptation to the individual's personal environment and the health care environment.

> *"Human systems have thinking and feeling capacities, rooted in consciousness and meaning, by which they adjust effectively to changes in the environment and, in turn, affect the environment."*
>
> *—Marudhar & Josfeena, (2019, p. 283)*

To practice within a holistic framework, the APN can apply each mode of Roy's adaptation process to ensure people are valued and supported in their quest for health and wellness. Highlighting the positive and negative influences of an environment, whether personal or health care related, the APN can help the person balance achievement and challenges, such as rising health care costs.

Nursing and the High Cost of Health Care: Meleis's Transition Theory

Major efforts to lower health care expenditure by applying economic principles such as fundholding, limiting services, capping or bundling payments, lean management, or pay-for-performance incentives have been tried in various jurisdictions; evaluations of these interventions on overall financial burden on society and/or patient/population health outcomes remain limited and unconvincing (Sturmberg & Bircher, 2019). Ideas to counter these

TABLE 8.3 Integrating Roy's Adaptive Modes to APN Practice Role in Assisting People's Journey to Health and Wellness Amid Rising Health Care Costs

Roy's Adaptive Modes	APN Clinician	APN Leader	APN Educator
Interdependence Mode	Strengthen relations between provider and patient by extending respect and valuing individual needs and health goals.	Ensure accessibility to department resources to support staff and colleague practice.	Build and reinforce a strong curricular framework to enhance and support student capabilities and skill acquisitions.
Physiologic-physical Mode	Be attentive in addressing physical needs.	Be attentive in addressing stress/burnout among staff and colleagues.	Be attentive in using a student-centered approach to education.
Role Function Mode	Be inquisitive in assessing the person's role in society and their social values.	Be inquisitive in assessing staff and colleague roles to understand workplace values.	Be inquisitive in assessing student role socialization to that of the professional nurse.
Self-Concept Group Identity Mode	Have genuine interest in assessing and understanding the person's integrity and self-perception(s).	Support interpersonal relationships among staff and colleagues to assess values and the mission of the unit.	Develop and support a learning environment that promotes role development (socialization).

ineffective initiatives have been studied, such as applying complex adaptive systems (CAS). However, the health care arena has seen more complications to establish an efficient system due to the pandemic effect. Nursing continues to be a central figure (influencer) in the equation and has the potential to offer innovation during a time of frustration and financial challenges.

APNs are required to expand their knowledge of the health care environment to provide holistic and appropriate care interventions. APNs are fundamental points of access to influence people, families, and communities. As nursing has established itself as a distinctive contributor to health care, APNs can further the profession by addressing major contributors to health care challenges, such as rising costs. A substantive and summative description of nursing was offered by Flaskerud and Halloran (1980), as "nurses manage the interaction between the patient and the environment to promote health or healing" (p. 4). One should inquire about the challenges faced in seeking health care. APNs are a pivotal part of identifying, assessing, addressing, and creating innovative solutions to support patients, staff, colleagues, and students' journey in receiving health care benefits while minimizing the burdens associated with health care costs.

> *"21st Century nursing is the glue that holds a patient's health care journey together." (What Is Nursing & What Do Nurses Do? | ANA Enterprise, 2017)*

APNs share expert knowledge and care experiences with health care systems by supporting and integrating a value-based model. From frontline nurses to APNs, nurses are advocates for minimizing waste. Nurses and APNs have demonstrated support for valuing certain initiatives within health care organizations, which ultimately can drive down cost. Initiatives, such as valuing teamwork and ensuring patients receive appropriate care through avenues such as optimized bundle payments and accountable care organizations (ACOs), promote preventative health, and inquire about patient challenges post-discharge such as SDOH. No matter the setting, nurses and APNs play a significant role in increasing efficiency, finding cost savings, and improving care center operating margins while being focused on achieving desired patient outcomes.

Afaf Ibrahim Meleis studied the concept of transitions, and the interventions that would assist people in making healthy transitions. At the individual and family levels, changes occurring in identities, roles, relationships, abilities, and patterns of behavior constitute transitions (Schumacher & Meleis, 1994). At the organizational level, transitional change occurs in structure, function, or dynamics (Schumacher & Meleis, 1994). According to Meleis et al. (2000), transition is complex and multidimensionally identified as awareness, engagement, change, difference, time span, critical points, and events. The APN can further delineate the causes and effects for health care costs from patients to systems at large.

> *"I believe very strongly that, while knowledge is universal, the agents for developing knowledge must reflect the nature of the questions that are framed and driven by the different disciplines about the health and well-being of individuals or populations."*
>
> —Meleis (2007, p. ix)

A major assumption of Meleis's transition theory is an individual's response to a transition is influenced by interactions with others. This reciprocal effect can lead to misunderstanding and misinformation regarding health care opportunities. Meleis's description of transitions can be viewed as the effect, whether the transition is healthy or unhealthy. Meleis describes the concept of transition conditions as facilitators and inhibitors, which are personal, community, and societal factors that mediate an individual's response to a transition (Meleis et al., 2000). As health care costs continue to impact people's choices, the possibility of transitioning to healthier lifestyles becomes less viable. An alignment of Meleis's transition conditions is viewed through the lens of the APN to create solutions for addressing the impact of rising health care costs. The conditions include developmental, situational, health-illness, and organizational transitions (Schumacher & Meleis, 1994).

TABLE 8.4 Meleis' Transition Conditions: Stimulating Innovative Response from APNs to Respond to High Healthcare Costs

Meleis's Transitional Conditions	Transitional Conditions Defined (Schumacher & Meleis, 1994)	APN Clinician	APN Leader	APN Educator
Developmental Transition	Focused on the individual's perspective during their response(s) of various stages throughout the life cycle	Providing resources for specific developmental transitions, such as parenthood and middle age, to address specific health needs during these life cycles with a proactive, preventative health focus	Recognizing individual staff needs based on changes through Benner's professional development from novice to expert and offering continuing educational resources to meet staff learning needs and the changing needs of patient demographics	Integrating the concept of developmental transitions to holistic health assessments promoting preventative health initiatives that are aligned to different developmental stages
Situational Transition	Changes in educational and professional roles	Embracing change in scope of practice for the APN clinician to engage in a broader role to influence policies and evaluations, leading to a VBC framework	Engaging staff who have completed different levels of educational degrees to be proactive in policy development and policy use, with a focus on VBC	Identifying and offering learning support for the student as each level of program is achieved, with a focus on student successful progression

TABLE 8.4 Meleis' Transition Conditions: Stimulating Innovative Response from APNs to Respond to High Healthcare Costs (*Continued*)

Meleis's Transitional Conditions	Transitional Conditions Defined (Schumacher & Meleis, 1994)	APN Clinician	APN Leader	APN Educator
Health-Illness Transition	Focused on how individuals experience illness and transition among levels of care	Assessing for individual transition during illness to find pathways to assist the individual to effective acceptance and illness management	Being active in the process and evaluation of patients transitioning from different levels of care, with a focus on care (case) management principles	Applying case management to teaching care interventions to highlight VBC goals and initiatives
Organizational Transition	"Changes in the wider social, political, or economic environment or by intraorganizational changes in structure or dynamics" (Schumacher & Meleis, 1994, p. 21)	Actively engaging in professional organizations to stay abreast of current changes and population needs while being an active voice for nursing with health care initiatives from institutional, system, state, and national levels	Embracing role as a change agent with a focus on encouraging team building and staff development to understand change and how to evaluate for effectiveness and efficiency standards	Integrating current health care challenges into teaching and learning activities to engage student thinking to that of a critical thinker regarding how to voice nursing knowledge, ethical standards, and innovation to practice and professional role development

Environment and the High Cost of Health Care: Ray's Theory of Bureaucratic Caring

As clinical settings have changed and grown since the pandemic, the opportunities for nursing to advance nursing science have also expanded. To take the environment at face value is to underestimate the meaning and impact this domain can have on overall health. The environment, per the lens of the nursing metaparadigm, can have many domains, from as the individual's physical environment to the individual's spiritual environment. Just as the person extends to family, social structures, and communities, the environment can be vast and a prospect for APNs to address influencing factors on the health and wellness of the person and a system. These factors can and should be grounded in spiritual, ethical, political, economic, legal, technological, educational, physical, and sociocultural dimensions.

APNs hold an important role in decreasing demands of multiple environmental factors to ensure patient, staff, and student experiences are authentic and effective. APN practice, whether it is focused on patient care, staff management, or student learning, should embed all environmental factors into each activity of the APN; therefore, nursing and the environment are viewed as complements.

For more information and to explore the domain of environment as it relates to nursing practice, please read the following article:

Bender, M., & Feldman, M. S. (2015). A practice theory approach to understanding the interdependency of nursing practice and the environment. *Advances in Nursing Science, 38*(2), 96–109. https://doi.org/10.1097/ans.0000000000000068

As the APN practices in multiple settings, a shared goal of cost savings is typically a major initiative. APNs can connect members of health care and educational systems to identify cost savings, improve efficiencies, and ultimately deliver appropriate nursing practice. The opportunities to offer fiscally enhanced performance must be grounded in a continued commitment to holistic practice in that all domains of the environment are assessed and acknowledged when planning care, leadership, and educational interventions. The reality is APNs are vital to care coordination, leadership initiatives, and educational strategies.

> *"Understanding and changing the emerging corporate culture of the health care system to benefit humankind is the most critical issue facing nursing educators, administrators, and practitioners."*
>
> *—Ray (1989, p. 31)*

As nurses and APNs navigate changing complexities within health care structures, organizational culture can have a large effect on nursing practice (or choices within the domain of the nurse's role). The environment within different health care systems and settings can have a major impact on the nurses and APNs, from intention of caring to implementation of caring interventions, potentially influencing the cost of care. Marilyn Ray's theory of bureaucratic caring addresses the environment in which caring is being determined and received. With Ray's theory, APNs can be guided to not only understand but to determine how the environment in which they are practicing can inhibit or promote spiritual-ethical caring that recognizes political, legal, economic, technological, educational, and sociocultural stimuli.

For more exploration on the use of Ray's theory of bureaucratic caring from the perspective of a nurse manager, please read the following article:

Lusiyana, A., Yetti, K., & Kuntarti, K. (2019). The strategies of bureaucratic caring implementation by nurse manager: A systematic review. *Enfermería Clínica, 29*(2), 41–46. https://doi.org/10.1016/j.enfcli.2019.05.003

A major premise of Ray's (1989) theory of bureaucratic caring is the concept of differential caring as it relates to role differentiation and work unit experiences in the complex organization of clinical (practice) settings. From Ray's research, economic, political, legal, and technological dimensions of caring were dominant to the social, ethical/spiritual dimensions. Overall, the theory revealed that the meaning of nursing and caring is not only transpersonal but also contextual, in other words, influenced by the social structure of complex organizations (the value system of a bureaucracy and humanistic caring). Figure 8.3 demonstrates the interconnectedness of

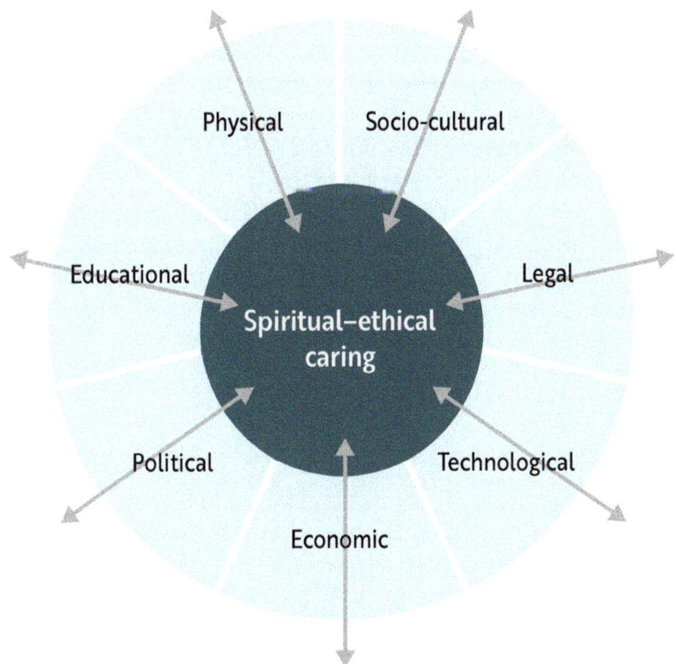

FIGURE 8.3 Ray's holographic theory of bureaucratic caring.

concepts; each part has meaning but makes an impact on how nurses and APNs provide spiritual-ethical caring.

Reflection on the nursing metaparadigm reminds us of how nursing interacts with specific phenomena. The environment is a major influence in caring practices. Ray (1989) compares change in complex organizations with a creative process and challenges nurses to step back and renew their perceptions of everyday events, to discover the embedded meanings, especially during organizational change. Using this practice, APNs can adapt and be innovative in care decisions as well as decisions regarding cost savings for the person and the system with a unifying approach. APNs can demonstrate aligned care, with each factor affecting the environment of a person and the setting in which care is being received and respond with more confidence to economic issues and be a valued member of the system as a contributor to health care economic stability.

As health care economics becomes more complex and costly, APNs can be a valued partner in their perceptions (experiences) of how care impacts financial gains (or strains). Changing policies drive financial trajectories. APNs can assist by engaging in a more comprehensive relationship with the patient, staff member, and student. Understanding major concepts such as uncertainty, adaptation, transition, and bureaucratic caring (differential caring) can be a launching point for engagement and innovation.

Figure Credits

Fig. 8.1: Statista, "Forecasted U.S. National Health Expenditure from 2021 to 2031 (in billion U.S. dollars)," https://www.statista.com/statistics/934283/total-us-national-health-expenditure-projection/. Copyright © 2024 by Statista.

Fig. 8.2: KFF, "Half of Adults Say It Is Difficult to Afford Health Care Costs, Including Large Shares of the Uninsured, Black, and Hispanic Adults, and Those with Lower Incomes," https://www.kff.org/health-costs/issue-brief/americans-challenges-with-health-care-costs/. Copyright © 2023 by KFF.

Fig. 8.3: Marilyn Ray, "Ray's Holographic Theory of Bureaucratic Caring," Nursing Administration Quarterly, vol. 13, no. 2. Copyright © 1989 by Lippincott Williams & Wilkins Inc.

CHAPTER 9

Aligning Theory to Poor Patient Outcomes

Key Terms

Assurance: A statement that something will certainly be true or will certainly happen, particularly when there has been doubt about it (Oxford Advanced Learner's Dictionary, n.d.).

Burnout: Unmanaged, chronic workplace stress resulting in mental and physical exhaustion, mental distance from the job, cynicism about the job, and reduced efficacy in the workplace (WHO, 2019).

Digital divide: An unequal access to digital technology, including smartphones, tablets, laptops, and the internet creating a division and inequality around access to information and resources (Wikipedia, 2023).

Health: A state of complete physical, mental, and social well-being and not merely the absence of disease or infirmity (WHO, n.d.).

Patient experience: Encompasses the range of interactions that patients have with the health care system, including their care from health plans and from doctors, nurses, and staff in hospitals, physician practices, and other health care facilities (Agency for Healthcare Research and Quality, n.d.).

Value: Health outcomes achieved that matter to patients relative to the cost of achieving those outcomes (Porter & Lee, 2013).

Vulnerable population: Patients who are racial or ethnic minorities, children, elderly, socioeconomically disadvantaged, underinsured, or with certain medical conditions who often have health conditions that are exacerbated by unnecessarily inadequate health care (Waisel, 2013).

Well-being: How people feel and how they function, both on a personal and a social level, and how they evaluate their lives as a whole (Mental Health Foundation, n.d.).

Introduction

To define patient outcomes is to describe attributes of the concept, which include the patient's functional status, patient safety, and patient satisfaction. This three-pronged view serves as a critical framework for the APN to deliver care, influence policy, and educate. Health care providers have been part of the analysis of patient outcomes as core measures in assessing a system's cost-effectiveness and quality care key indicators.

Patient outcomes are influenced by many factors, such as access to health care, socioeconomic status, and level of education, to name a few; however, looking through the lens of the nursing profession, one would be remiss to not recognize the impact of the pandemic on the nursing workforce. As nurses continue to make up the largest segment of the U.S. health care workforce in the post-pandemic era, nurses remain essential providers of quality and safe patient care. The pandemic uncovered more of the burdens placed on nurses, such as the persistence of understaffing, which lead to an increase in nurse-reported stress and burnout. The concerns related to the impact of burnout among nurses can be felt by all health care systems in the United States. Results from a 2020 survey indicate that almost two thirds of nurses (62%) experience burnout, especially with nurses under 65 (69%; ANA, 2022). A 2021 integrative review examining the pre- and post-COVID-19 pandemic literature on nursing turnover found that since the pandemic's onset, there has been a significant increase in nurse turnover intention (Falatah, 2021). Nurses reported high levels of emotional exhaustion, depersonalization, and reduced feelings of personal accomplishment (Galanis et al., 2021). As nurses changed practice settings or left the profession, poor patient outcomes increased.

The pandemic instilled fear. Through fear, many people refrained from accessing health care services. From screenings to management of chronic diseases, these gaps in care caused many people to suffer complications to their health and well-being. Telehealth became a lifeline to reach patients and continue the work needed to care for and provide health care services, yet persistent needs of patients linger and burden an already diminished health care system. Despite the innovations of technology to assist in health care, many people continue to suffer from a widening gap of services to assess, treat, and educate on living a well life. SDOH have taken on new meaning since the pandemic. COVID-19 disproportionality affected vulnerable populations. All have felt the impacts of COVID from economic, social, and educational fronts. The pandemic magnified vulnerable populations by exposing inequality gaps, particularly on physical, socioeconomic, and mental well-being.

Vulnerable populations continue to be impacted by the health care gap resulting from income, employment, accessibility, food insecurity, and digital divide factors. Groups nurses need to assess that may face additional challenges in enduring the effects of the pandemic are mothers and children, older adults, persons with disabilities, and low-income individuals and families. Key indicators of vulnerability include but are not limited to the following:

- Low income: Lack of access the health care and live in environments not conducive to good health
- Age: The very old and the very young
- Race and ethnicity: Higher correlations to low income
- Undereducated
- People living with disabilities
- Limited English proficiency
- Homeless
- Uninsured
- LGBTQIA

In addition, natural and manmade disasters are factors that worsen communities' health, creating insecurity with basic necessities, such as shelter and food. The changing landscapes and impact of disasters have lingering effects on the health of many, particularly vulnerable populations.

CDC/Agency for Toxic Substances and Disease Registry Social Vulnerability Index

For more information on vulnerable populations' risks before, during, and after disasters, please review the Social Vulnerability Index, which provides potential negative effects on communities caused by external stresses on human health.

https://www.atsdr.cdc.gov/placeandhealth/svi/index.html

Improving health outcomes by addressing SDOH can transform lives and people's ability to reach personalized levels of health-related goals. APNs are key in ensuring all people can be given the opportunity to achieve wellness. Despite the impacts of the pandemic and the growing challenges within health care systems across the country, improved patient outcomes must remain a pivotal target for health care initiatives and for the education of current and future health care providers.

This chapter will explore the following learning objectives in relation to poor patient outcomes.

1. Explore the nursing metaparadigm through the challenges set forth post-pandemic on poor outcomes in patient pursuit to health and wellness.
2. Align selected nursing theories and models to each domain of the nursing metaparadigm: health, person, nurse, and environment.
3. Analyze the role of APN clinician, leader, and educator to address poor patient outcomes to apply clinical specialty skills through nursing theory to assist patient pursuits to health and wellness.

Nursing Metaparadigm: Addressing Poor Patient Outcomes

Quality care is a key indicator of good health care. To have good health care is to have improved patient outcomes. The nursing metaparadigm can serve as a framework for addressing the multifaceted influences that lead to poor patient outcomes, whether those outcomes are an increase in mortality across the life span or rising chronic disease–related hospital admissions. The metaparadigm serves to organize nurses' care delivery and is inexplicitly linked to patients and their health. Nursing is clearly aware of the impact a patient's physical and social environment has on their unique experiences of health. Benner (2012) called for the environment to be distinct and therefore not limiting its scope for the nurse in practice. An environment can be defined in many ways and has fluidity to change throughout an individual's lifetime. By expanding the concept of environment, the APN can study, assess, and evaluate nursing knowledge related to new caring environments, especially the environment in which the nurse and patient build a relationship, and hence influence patient outcomes.

As the pandemic has redefined what health is for many, the APN can be a conduit to improving health care delivery to ensure health goals are reached, maintained, and adapted to the environments that impact each patient. Part of this process to employ quality, safe care while implementing value-driven principles is to engage the patient to be center of their health care journey. Taking on health and wellness initiatives through self-empowerment or independence is highly beneficial. Each domain of patient outcomes (patient's functional status, patient safety, and patient satisfaction) supports an active plan toward a complete state of physical, mental, and social well-being, or health.

Health and Poor Patient Outcomes: Roper, Logan, and Tierney's Model for Nursing Based on a Model of Living

Health (nursing metaparadigm), patient outcomes, and value-based care intersect and have a symbiotic relationship. Exploring each as a separate concept would limit their contributions to quality, safe care. VBC can hold multiple meanings, including cost-effectiveness, best practices, and patient satisfaction. Because patient outcomes are a critical element of patient satisfaction and cost-effective care, the APN plays a prominent role in strategizing solutions and innovations to create an environment that upholds health as a fundamental dimension in measuring today's health care systems.

Simply having knowledge related to health care assurance and other SDOH influences on patient outcomes is ineffective for performing in the health care system. Every level of health care, from education to practice, to policy development, must be done with a central goal to create value-based, equitable care. Missed opportunities to address each layer of health can pose risks resulting in poor and unwanted outcomes for patients. The APN can innovate through nursing theories and models to address these by considering multiple patient environments and inspiring patient independence.

Patient independence is a highly important factor relating to physical and mental well-being. This assumption can be easily transferred and seen through the lens of an elderly patient. Having choices, feeling empowered, and personalizing health needs creates many opportunities for the APN to assist patients in planning care, which focuses on healthier patient outcomes.

Roper, Logan, and Tierney's model for nursing based on a model of living evaluates a person's daily life. Under the assumptions of this theory, the APN can view the changes a patient is facing as a result of illness by planning to rebuild patient independence. Each influential patient environment, such as family life, social life, physical shelter, and even the health care environment, is assessed for interventions to support independence, especially areas in which it may be difficult for the patient to acknowledge, such as performing activities of daily living. A key to this theory is understanding that with each health care event the patient should be provided opportunity and resources to reach their individualized, maximum potential for independence.

The theoretical assumptions of Roper, Logan, and Tierney's model for nursing based on a model of living correlates with other nursing theories, such as Virginia Henderson's needs theory. An emphasis is placed on achievements of health by addressing activities like sleeping, breathing, eating, and physical movement. The model of living takes a holistic view. Each person's need requires a comprehensive assessment. Roper's theory values independence through biological, sociocultural, environmental, political and economic factors. APNs can integrate assumptions found in Roper's theory to assist patients in gaining independence and generating increased patient satisfaction and improved health.

TABLE 9.1 Adoption of Roper, Logan, and Tierney's Model for Nursing Based on a Model of Living for the APN in Practice: Enhancing Independence for Improved Patient Outcomes

Roper's Model of Living Independence Factors	Description	APN Clinician	APN Leader	APN Educator
Biological	Addresses the impact of the overall health, of current injury or illness and the scope of the patient's anatomy and physiology	Emphasis on assessing patient ability to perform activities of daily living by means of physiological adaptation and reaching/maintaining independence	Testing nursing assessment processes in various clinical and nonclinical settings to address biological deficits and adaptations to meet activities of daily living	Considering research and testing of nursing frameworks within an educational platform and evaluating systematic and holistic physiologic patient assessments focused on functioning and ability to meet required activities of daily living
Psychological	Addresses the impact of emotion, cognition, and spiritual beliefs	Recognizes and employs assessments of patient psychological reactions to deficits in activities of daily living with incorporation of interventions that the patient needs to know, think, hope, feel, and believe to maintain or regain independence	Employs systematic policies and procedures to nursing practice from a holistic lens, incorporating the need to understand patient emotional, spiritual, and cognitive thinking (beliefs) as a testable framework to evaluate patient satisfaction and improve outcomes	Integrating curriculum that understands the assessment of independence as a factor of patient outcomes in that emotions, thoughts, and beliefs are opportunities for nursing assessment and focused interventions

TABLE 9.1 Adoption of Roper, Logan, and Tierney's Model for Nursing Based on a Model of Living for the APN in Practice: Enhancing Independence for Improved Patient Outcomes (*Continued*)

Roper's Model of Living Independence Factors	Description	APN Clinician	APN Leader	APN Educator
Sociocultural	Addresses society and culture as influences on patient expectations of achieving and maintaining independence	Assesses both perceptions and social and cultural contexts for patient completing activities of daily living in a safe manner	Acknowledges the social and cultural perceptions of independence and the value of using resources to achieve/assist/support maintaining or readapting activities of daily living	Provides learning growth and opportunities to evaluate the effects of social and cultural influences on patient independence and health maintenance
Environmental	Addresses a reciprocal relationship between environmental factors and the ability to adapt and maintain independence through activities of daily living	Acknowledges the impact of activities of daily living on the environment and how the environment can support or hinder patient independence	Promotes use of environmental resources to support staff interventions to achieve patient independence with less waste of resources using a "green" concept to utilizing environmental resources and influences on patient independence	Instructs through a curriculum that promotes an efficient use of the environment and resources to support the patient's maintenance and adaptation of independence
Politico Economical	Addresses funding and benefits from an economic and political viewpoint on achievement of patient independence	Advocates for programs and resources to aid patients in achieving independence	Lobbies and drafts support for funding, policies, programs, and reforms to promote interventions supporting patient independence	Integrates curriculum political and economic factors that support interventions and resources necessary to assist nurses in planning care and interventions

Person and Poor Patient Outcomes: Henderson's Nursing Need Theory

Persons (patients) are complex and have a multitude of factors that influence their trajectories toward health and wellness. Health outcomes are not stagnant and will fluctuate over a person's lifetime. Patient outcomes are often viewed as stand-alone data when used to measure quality care through a cost-effective lens. APNs are aware of the shifting dimensions of a person and are in tune with assessing these changes. Poor patient outcomes are not meant to be a singular data point; rather, the APN can guide, inspire, and educate toward improved health and well-being.

Often, patient satisfaction is recorded and assessed for quality care measures; however, the data retrieved from these types of surveys may not tell the wholes story, or the patient experience. By using the nursing metaparadigm and evaluating poor patient outcomes, the APN can benefit from assessing the latter. Patient experience, according to the Agency for Healthcare Research and Quality (n.d.), appeals to the health care provider to find out from patients if something that should happen in a health care setting (e.g., clear communication with a provider) actually happened or how often it happened.

Most health care systems' mission is to provide patient-centered care (PCC), yet patient outcomes demonstrate a contrasting view. PCC should foster quality improvements, creating a contract between the health care system and the person(s) to be accountable to the people they serve (Larson et al., 2019). The Lancet Global Health Commission on High-Quality Health Systems in the SDG define quality care as care that is effective in maintaining or improving health and is person centered, meaning that it is respectful of and responsive to individual preferences, needs, and values (Larson et al., 2019). Studies have demonstrated PPC is associated with increased health care utilization and improved health outcomes (Doyle et al., 2013). Understanding the nuances to concepts such as patient experience places the APN in a position to enhance skills that promote PCC, and thus quality care. By engaging in deductive thinking, the APN improves patient outcomes.

Similar to Roper's model of living, Henderson's need theory focuses on independence to support progression toward health and wellness goals. Due to its wide usability and application, the theory's assumptions align well with PCC and improving health outcomes. Henderson also used deductive reasoning as a premise in that actions are based on inquiries and solutions. The theory follows the primary assumption that an individual achieves wholeness by maintaining physiological and emotional balance (Henderson, 1966). While there is an alignment of Henderson's 14 needs to Maslow's

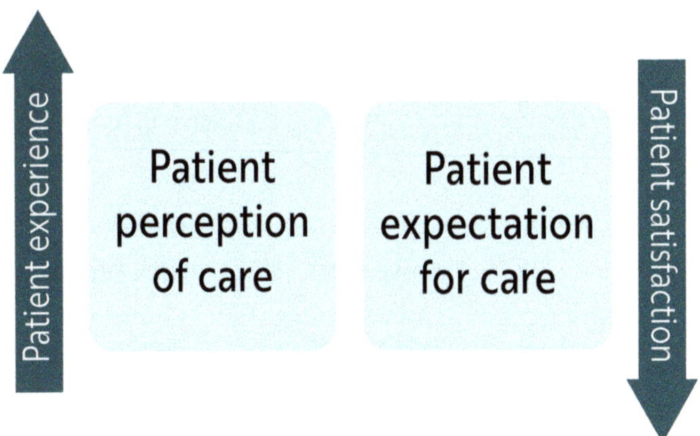

FIGURE 9.1 Contrasting patient experience with patient satisfaction.

hierarchy of needs, the Henderson's theory represents the activities required in attaining not just survival but good health.

To gain independence the nurse must recognize the necessity to empower patients to accept and adapt to health situations. Even through a new medical condition (diagnosis), a person can adapt to maintain independence and self-care. Henderson's theory provides a logical and sequential framework for the nurse and APN to employ in various clinical settings while caring for the person as a sum of biopsychosocial needs and not a condition or consumer of a product. Henderson's theory brings nursing back to holism and the practice of PCC, which evidence has proven leads to healthier outcomes for patients.

Case Study: Integrating Henderson's Need Theory to Enhance Independence and Outcomes

Case Scenario

Ms. Y is a 22-year-old female client admitted to the surgical unit post-suicide attempt by ingesting antifreeze. Ms. Y's mother reports Ms. Y was due to be married in 1 week and had no clear idea why Ms. Y would try to take her life. Ms. Y lived with her fiancée for 2 years and at times was reported, by family members, to have highs and lows, resulting in numerous break-ups with her fiancée.

Ms. Y's physical assessment revealed an alert and oriented depressed female. Her chief complaint was difficulty breathing, and her CT scan and endoscopy revealed significant damage to her larynx and oral mucosa, as well as developing stomach ulcers. A liquid diet was prescribed; however, Ms. Y disliked the taste and refused to eat. A Foley catheter was placed to monitor her input and output. Within 2 days, Ms. Y showed signs of dehydration as evidenced by dry membranes, tenting of the

(continued)

skin, sunken eyes, and dark, amber-colored urine. Ms. Y became a safety risk as her ambulation demonstrated imbalance of gait. Ms. Y denied participation in hygiene practices and refused to speak to interdisciplinary team members.

Application of Henderson's Need Theory Through APN roles

APN Clinician	APN Leader	APN Educator
Conduct a close assessment of the 14 needs to determine short- and long-term comprehensive plans of care with an awareness of an acute crisis situation from a holistic view: biopsychosocial. Lack of independence has a direct impact on patient outcomes, requiring interventions from health care providers to ensure adequate resources to meet the patient's mind, body, and spiritual needs.	Ensure nursing staff have the resources and knowledge to address patient needs through a systematic and holistic approach. Advocate and lead policy development to promote plans of care that address patient independence from admission through discharge.	Educate students on the value of patient independence and the relationship to health and improved patient outcomes. Incorporate holistic assessment skills into educational curricula and ongoing nursing professional development activities.

Nursing and Poor Patient Outcomes: Benner's Novice to Expert Theory

Nursing holds an influential role in patient outcomes. Nurses are advocates and essential in preventing patient deterioration and adverse events (medication errors and infection). According to a report by the *Cochrane Review*, nurses (both RNs and APNs) can effectively expand the capacity of the primary care workforce; qualified nurses can probably provide equal or better quality of care compared to primary care doctors (Laurant et al., 2018). In addition, the review found that nurses achieve higher levels of patient satisfaction compared to primary care doctors and that patients are slightly more likely to attend follow-up appointments with nurses than with doctors (Laurant et al., 2018). Despite the challenges facing the nursing workforce, such as staffing and retention, the future for nursing is bright and can make a great impact on patient health.

> *"This review shows that for some ongoing and urgent physical complaints and for chronic conditions, trained nurses, such as nurse practitioners, practice nurses, and registered nurses, probably provide equal or possibly even better quality of care compared to primary care doctors, and probably achieve equal or better health outcomes for patients."*
>
> *—Laurant et al. (2018, para. 7)*

The level of clinical knowledge and judgment cannot be undervalued or dismissed. APNs have increased scopes of practice and expertise to add wider safety nets for patients to receive care focused on healing, adaptation, learning, and rehabilitation. The nurse–patient relationship is a dynamic factor impacting the patient experience. Studies have shown a good nurse–patient relationship reduces the number of days a patient spends in a hospital setting (Molina-Mula & Gallo-Estrada, 2020). The nurse acts as a resource and advocate, allowing the patient the autonomy to make decisions affecting their health and wellness. The health and well-being of the nurse must also be taken into consideration as a correlation between nurse satisfaction and patient outcomes has been a belief in health care for a long time.

With the increasing demands for quality assurance and quality improvement standards, the APN acquires skills and knowledge appropriate for addressing domains within the patient experience, such as SDOH, low socioeconomic status, health literacy, and cultural awareness. Working within these domains, the APN gains key skills. Communication, clinical judgment, collaboration, organization, assessment, evaluation, case management, and teaching are just a few of the expanding skills for the APN to achieve in order to function at an optimal level impacting patient outcomes. The dynamic challenges in the health care system APNs face requires an active response to engage in skill development and expertise.

Benner's novice to expert nursing theory guides the nurse through a continuum of professional growth. Knowledge learned, from a new graduate to years of nursing practice, accumulate to inform the APN in practice. Acknowledging that a nursing career is fluid and adaptive gives the nurse the opportunity to expand and become flexible in practice. A foundation to Benner's theory falls within the principles of experiential learning. Through experiences, reflection, and learning, the APN builds competencies, expertise, and ethical comportment. Benner's theory empowers the APN to continue to grow within the profession and specialty and beyond their educational degree.

Aligning to the Dreyfus (1982) model of skill acquisition, Benner proposes expert practice is holistic and situational. A noteworthy premise to Benner's theory is that the nurse will fluctuate from novice to expert throughout their career. Even an experienced nurse in a new clinical situation can make an incorrect or inaccurate response in practice. Through this process of nursing development, the APN utilizes reflection to gain interpretation of missed or incorrect actions, opening pathways to explore alternatives in any given situation. The prerequisite of expert-level nursing is reflective practice, or metacognition, leading to innovative interventions to maximize patient experiences and outcomes. As the APN cycles through Benner's novice to expert, the concept of individualized nursing care emerges.

Individualized nursing care is considered an indicator for quality care to enhance patient outcomes (Papastavrou et al., 2015). Individualized care constitutes the basis of the holistic philosophy, values, and ethical codes of nursing and includes planning and practicing nursing care in accordance with the individual characteristics, requirements, preferences, experiences, feelings, perceptions, and opinions of the individual and incorporating the individual to this process (Papastavrou et al., 2015). Attention to holistic nursing care principles in the nurse–patient relationship enhances prospects for care, which is perceived by the patient as valuable and responsive to individual needs.

As individualized nursing care is built on experience, or experiential learning, situational meaning is gained. An expert nurse's practice will flourish when the expert nurse values and practices consistent reflection. The expert nurse will test innovations and refine interventions through theoretical and practical knowledge. Promoting expert nurses to forge forward and not stand still is critical to impacting patient outcomes. Individualized nursing care through the actions of the expert nurse grows nursing knowledge for all levels of nurses, creating a web of innovation, research, evidence, best practice, and mutual support.

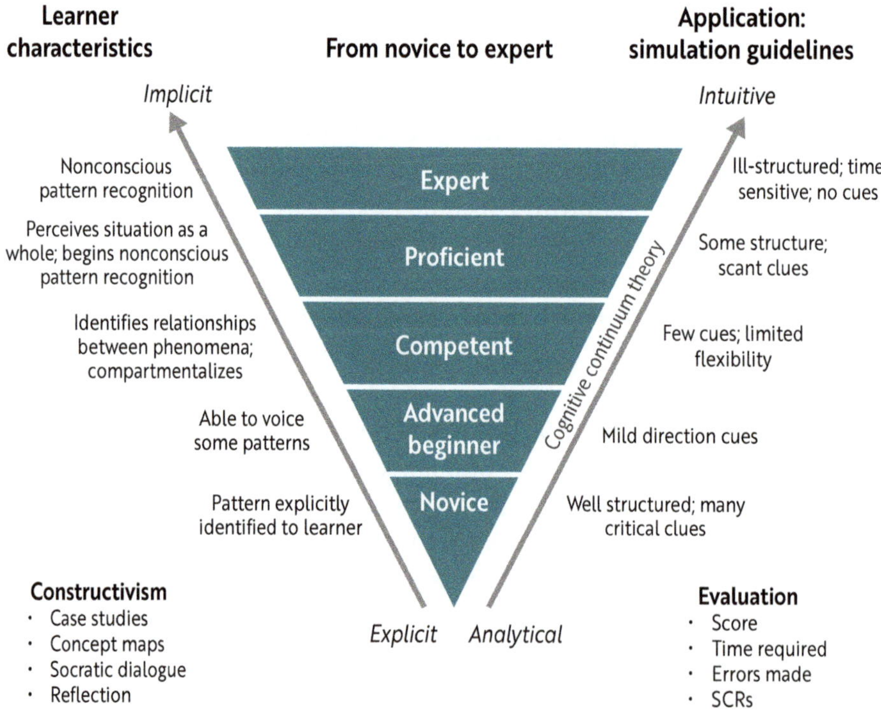

FIGURE 9.2 Valuing the continuum of Benner's novice to expert theory for the APN.

Environment and Poor Patient Outcomes: Nightingale's Environmental Theory

Environment is multifactorial when addressing patient outcomes. The environments (social, cultural, or physical) will vary in the influence on patients' health and wellness. Having low income and lack of access to health care services prevents individuals from reaching good health. Good health is a subjective concept yet is often described beyond functional status to also include meaning and making an impact on others. The cycle of poverty demonstrates the negative and poor outcomes experienced by those living in these constraints of good health.

The all-encompassing effects of the environment place roadblocks on a patient's health journey. Nursing can look to Maslow and Henderson to assess the basic needs of living, which leads to a sense of security and safety, but the environment is a broad concept that has complex meanings and controls on patient health. The environment can produce interactions among others and subsequently create social support or remove it. A social network is often quantified or defined by individuals' perceptions of social capital. In today's social environment, this can be the number of likes on a social network posting. A person can also perceive the nurse as social support; however, post discharge the patient would be left without a structure that extends into a more personal realm. Moreover, the quality of relationships may be misperceived, leading to lost use of needed resources. The environment can induce motivation to act or change behavior. The environment can influence mood (feelings/emotions). As one struggles to obtain housing or clean air and water, the cycle of depression accelerates, with little to no room for valuing and accepting health-forward interventions. In today's health care environment, the concept built environment is extensively studied for its effects on healing and the patient health care experience. Yet, Nightingale provides nursing with a systems model with the patient at the center of their surroundings, both physical and social, so as to not lose sight of holistic care practices.

When one thinks of Nightingale, one thinks of the term *environment*. Nightingale pioneered numerous beliefs and practices throughout nursing's professional journey and remains as relevant today as during the Crimean War. Nursing and health care alike were summoned to Nightingale's theoretical principles during the COVID pandemic. As a forerunner to germ theory, Nightingale acutely understood the essential need for sanitation and infection reduction through a clean environment. As impressive as Nightingale's early work was during wartime efforts, her contributions to how nursing views the environment is far more comprehensive than on face value.

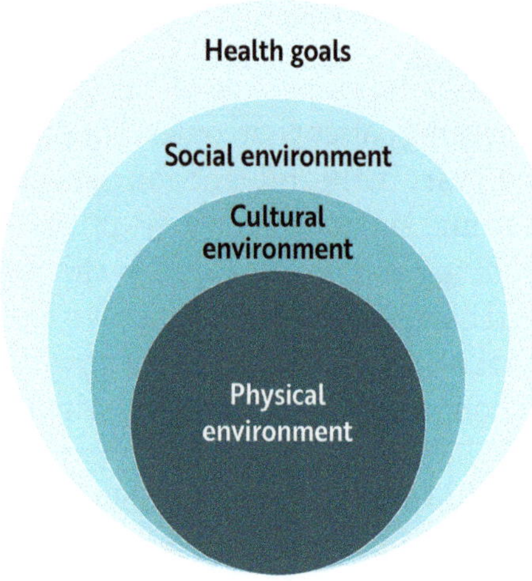

FIGURE 9.3 In pursuit of good health: Relationship of environments and achievement of health goals.

Nightingale's (1980) definition of the *environment* includes anything, through manipulation, that assists in putting the individual in the best possible condition for nature to act. Within the view of Nightingale's environment, the APN will include all types of environments that impact a patient's perceptions, actions, and reactions regarding health and well-being. Maintaining the patient, staff member, and student at the center will promote the APN to ensure a person-centered care approach while assessing all environments that influence a patient's ability to reach health goals.

Figure Credit

Fig. 9.2: Parkhide Hassani, Alireza Abdi, Rostam Jalali, and Nader Salari, "Valuing the Continuum of Benner's Novice to Expert Theory for the APN," International Journal of Evidence-Based Healthcare, vol. 15, no. 4. Copyright © 2017 by John Wiley & Sons, Inc.

CHAPTER 10

Aligning Theory to Unmask Health Care Disparities

Key Terms

Advocacy: Activities in which health care organizations work with partner social care organizations to promote policies that facilitate the creation and redeployment of assets or resources to address health and social needs (National Academies of Sciences, Engineering, and Medicine, 2019).

Alignment: Activities undertaken by health care systems to understand existing social care assets in the community, organize them to facilitate synergies, and invest in and deploy them to positively affect health outcomes (National Academies of Sciences, Engineering, and Medicine, 2019).

Assistance: Activities that reduce social risk by aiding in connecting patients with relevant social care resources (National Academies of Sciences, Engineering, and Medicine, 2019).

Awareness: Activities that identify the social risks and assets of defined patients and populations (National Academies of Sciences, Engineering, and Medicine, 2019).

Culturally congruent care: Means to provide care that are meaningful and fit with cultural beliefs and lifeways (Leininger, 1999).

Dwelling: A phenomenological concept, refers to a fundamental atmosphere of having a foothold in existence, that is, a sense of belonging, being safe, and feeling at home (Martinsen, 2006).

Health disparities: A particular type of health difference that is closely linked with social, economic, and/or environmental disadvantage (Healthy People 2030, n.d.).

Health equity: The attainment of the highest level of health for all people (Healthy People 2030, n.d.).

Synergy (model): A conceptual framework that aligns patient needs with nurse competencies (American Association of Critical Care Nurses, n.d.).

Transcultural nursing: Various culture-related aspects of health care delivery that can affect disease management and the status of individuals' health and well-being (Leininger, 2002).

Introduction

Prior to assessing or applying theory or models of practice to address health disparities within the health care and educational environments, it is essential to understand specific terminology. *Health disparities* has been widely defined as a particular health difference that is closely linked with economic, social, and/or environmental disadvantage(s) (Healthy People 2030, n.d.). Closely associated is the term *health equity*. Healthy People 2030 (n.d.) defines *health equity* as the attainment of the highest level of health for all people by valuing each individual equally. Root causes of many health disparities lie in SDOH, which include groups of people who systematically experience greater obstacles to health based on their race or ethnicity, religion, socioeconomic status, gender, age, and geographic location; mental health; cognitive, sensory, or physical disability; sexual orientation or gender identity; nationality or immigration status (Healthy People 2030, n.d.). Healthy People 2030 continues to reach for goals focused on eliminating health disparities and improving health for all populations. As leaders in health care, APNs can effectively influence reduction of health disparities to achieve health equity by being engaged in addressing root causes through individual, organizational, and policy levels. Examples include using effective communication skills based on individual comprehension during patient, staff and student encounters and on patient- (person) or student-centered approaches at various care levels (primary to tertiary) and interactions while additionally advocating for broader adoption of cultural and linguistically appropriate service (CLAS) standards. Other advocacy initiatives include lobbying for broader scope of practice for the APN clinician for all states while valuing the expertise of APN leaders and educators for contributions at staff and student levels, hence influencing the current and future nursing workforce.

For more information on the CLAS standards, please use the following link:

- https://thinkculturalhealth.hhs.gov/clas

The W.K. Kellogg Foundation (2023) and the nonprofit Altarum reported racial health disparities result in $93 billion in excess medical care costs and $42 billion in lost productivity each year. Health disparities and inequities have persisted in U.S. health care; however, there is no doubt COVID-19 unveiled many layers of health disparities in the United States (and globally). Statistics have repeatedly confirmed the striking differences in mortality rates among those infected with COVID-19. Black and Hispanic individuals were three times were likely than White individuals to die from COVID-19 (Godoy, 2020). According to research by Penn Medicine, one in 10 Black people who died from COVID-19 would still be alive today if racial health disparities in hospital quality did not exist (Patient Engagement HIT, 2021). Nana-Sinkam et al. (2021) report the impact of COVID-19 and its spotlight on health disparities has created an impetus for reexamining the root causes within health care systems in the United States. A prioritized commitment to strategic partnerships between academic and nonacademic settings can be key to directing the required steps in understanding health disparities (Nana-Sinkam et al., 2021). While APNs can be instrumental in overseeing, steering, and supporting change in reducing health disparities, their own practice responses within their specialty roles, can be greatly influenced by the use of nursing theory to support a focused, holistic, and equitable care approach.

> *"Health is more than absence of disease; it is about economics, education, environment, empowerment, and community. The health and wellbeing of the people is critically dependent upon the health system that serves them. It must provide the best possible health with the least disparities and respond equally well to everyone."*
>
> *—Joycelyn Elders, Former U.S. Surgeon General*

This chapter will explore the following learning objectives in relation to poor patient outcomes:

1. Explore the nursing metaparadigm through the challenges set forth in post-pandemic health disparities.
2. Align selected nursing theories and models to each domain of the nursing metaparadigm: health, person, nurse, and environment.
3. Analyze the role of APN clinician, leader, and educator to address health disparities and to apply clinical specialty skills with nursing theory to assist patient pursuits toward health and wellness.

Nursing Metaparadigm: Addressing Health Disparities

"Health equity is achieved when everyone has a fair and just opportunity to be as healthy as possible" (NASEM, 2017a, p. 32). As many in our communities serve various roles, such as delivering goods, stocking shelves, processing foods, cleaning hospitals, and harvesting crops were identified as "essential" as a result of COVID-19 lockdowns, it is within these populations that health disparities exist. Longitudinal studies have defined low income as a prevalent link to those who do not receive adequate or timely health care. Consider the single parent who is working as a grocery clerk 40 hours a week and has no time to take off for being sick or to care for a sick child. As a result, the single parent has an immediate loss of income with a high risk of delayed health care. Even public health initiatives of primary prevention are often lost and underused due to the harmful effects associated with SDOH. As the nursing metaparadigm directs nursing actions through practice and research, it also reminds nurses of the importance of further phenomena that require nursing attention, such as decreasing poor health outcomes.

The *Integrating Social Care into the Delivery of Health Care* report identified five areas that can facilitate social care into health care: adjustment, assistance, alignment, advocacy, and awareness (NASEM, 2019). Each of the five areas can serve to assist the APN to address health inequities while aligning associated concepts to the nursing metaparadigm.

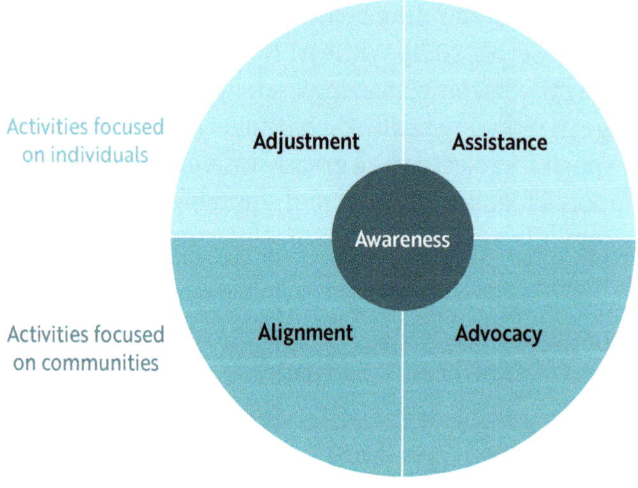

FIGURE 10.1 Areas of activity to strengthen integration of social care into health care (NASEM, 2019).

As APNs expand their knowledge and scope of practice, attention to underserved populations due to health disparities becomes an ethical obligation. By valuing a commitment to self-care and metacognition as tools to maintain a healthy and productive use of one's advanced nursing competences, the APN clinician, leader, and educator can offer a diverse and experiential approach to improving health equity. Although, one must not

TABLE 10.1 Distinguishing Five Activity Areas of Social Care Through the Lens of the APN and Nursing Metaparadigm

Social Care Activity	APN Clinician	APN Leader	APN Educator	Link to Nursing Metaparadigm
Awareness	Knowing population/demographics in which the APN clinician serves with identification of intentional or unintentional biases	Increasing knowledge of staff to understand various cultures/demographics of people served in their community	Integrating information of various demographics and SDOH in curricula to broaden student understanding of impacts to health	Person Environment
Adjustment	Proposal/integration of alternative sources of treatments, such as telehealth services, to widen the options of point of care contact	Enhance work environment by providing staff with more options to provide social care, such as meal or transportation vouchers	Engage students to use clinical judgment to adjust care to fulfill potential missed care opportunities through active learning modalities	Health Environment
Assistance	Integrate social care assessments to highlight at-risk or neglected basic necessities to enhance identification of resources needed	Collaborate in an innovative way through direct input from nursing staff to case management to link resources in a more efficient manner	Integrate resource assessments in student concept/care mapping	Nurse Environment
Alignment	Collaborate with health care administrators to invest in community stakeholders to highlight community/social resources	Empower staff to use community outreach as a means to establish health care provider and community relationships	Support student community engagement by incorporating volunteer and independent projects with community resources supporting the moral imperative to aid underserved populations	Nurse Person Environment

(Continued)

TABLE 10.1 Distinguishing Five Activity Areas of Social Care Through the Lens of the APN and Nursing Metaparadigm (*Continued*)

Social Care Activity	APN Clinician	APN Leader	APN Educator	Link to Nursing Metaparadigm
Advocacy	Lobby for policy change directed at the point of care to provide sufficient time and resources to address health inequities at the local, state, and federal levels	Lead change with policy that addresses patients' social needs during times of health care service	Include research on use of policy development and importance of advocacy to support policy acceptance to create change in health inequities	Nurse Person Health Environment

forget where nursing knowledge comes from and how it is connected to the human experience. The answer echoes the generalizability and usability of nursing theory.

Health and Unmasking Health Disparities: Leininger's Transcultural Nursing Theory

Health care disparities create chronic stressors. The human body is an incredible system with the ability to manage stressors with protective mechanisms. A low income, unsafe living conditions, food insecurity, abuse, and oppression lead to chronic stress and maladaptation. Chronic stress leads to changes in autoimmune, endocrine, and neurologic systems and has been linked to health conditions such as hypertension and preterm birth (Steptoe & Marmot, 2002). Health care disparities, often rooted in socioeconomic, racial, or ethnic factors, continue to persist (Sagar & Sagar, 2018).

These disparities lead to unequal access to quality care and poorer health outcomes among marginalized groups. When a patient's values and beliefs are aligned to how their health care is delivered, synergy is created, leading to satisfaction and congruence with individual needs. Yet, statistics, such as the rising maternal morbidity and mortality rates over the last 10 years in the United States (U.S. Department of Health and Human Services, 2022), elucidating health disparities are uncovered. Poor wages, lack of access to adequate health care, and language barriers are a few of the roadblocks many U.S. citizens face that result in poor health outcomes. The IOM's *Future of Nursing* report in 2010 identified the changing U.S. demographics calling for a more diverse nursing workforce to meet these challenges. Despite the strong call for changes in cultural care and a diverse nursing workforce,

> *"If human beings are to survive and live in a healthy, peaceful, and meaningful world, then nurses and other health care providers need to understand the cultural care beliefs, values, and lifeways of people in order to provide culturally congruent and beneficial health care."*
> —Leininger (1978, p. 3)

health disparities continue to increase, with a strong need for the entirety of the health care workforce to meet patient challenges with cultural knowledge and application of cultural competence. As statistics continue to be bleak and declines in health outcomes rise, nursing theory can be a starting point to address health disparities. Madeleine Leininger's transcultural nursing theory promotes cultural care as part of nursing's routine assessment with a focus on increasing patient compliance, healing, and wellness.

To begin discussing Madeleine Leininger's transcultural nursing theory, it is important to note its focus. Leininger's theory includes an emphasis on cultures, health, and nursing phenomena. Intuitive from the theory's assumptions is the concept of culturally congruent care. The basis of culturally congruent care includes active listening by the health care provider of individual perceptions, which then can transition to utilizing different care approaches and comprehensive follow-up care. As an anthropologist, Leininger understood the importance of recognizing, identifying, and applying cultural values into formulation of nursing care plans. Over time, as schools integrated Leininger's theoretical works on cultural care into curricula, other nursing associations embraced the concept of inclusive health care. In 2015, the ANA published standards of practice for cultural congruency. Cultural congruent care remains a standard of care and has formed the basic foundations of nursing practice. Despite the wide adoption of cultural care standards, a new approach to cultural care guided by theory can address patient values, individualize health needs, provide access to care, and create synergy between health care provider and patient.

Transcultural nursing holds a focus on cultural caring, health, and nursing phenomena. Leininger defines transcultural nursing as providing culture specific and universal nursing care practices for the health and well-being of people or to help them face unfavorable human conditions, illness, or death in culturally meaningful ways (Leininger & McFarland, 2002). According to Leininger and McFarland (2002), all nurses need to be prepared to serve vulnerable populations. By adopting Leininger and McFarland's proposal for nurses to view themselves as global citizens prepared to care in a culturally meaningful way to enhance health, each APN can make an impact from the levels of clinician, leader, and educator. APNs have opportunities to work with immigrants and a plethora of patients from various cultural backgrounds. By analyzing various cultural encounters and applying Leininger's transcultural caring theory, a systematic and competent approach to cultural care is practiced.

Application of Leininger's Transcultural Care Theory to Address Health Disparities Through the Lens of Health in the Nursing Metaparadigm

Scenario

A Mexican American woman is late to her appointment. The patient explained her situation: lack of transportation, single mother, limited income, childcare needs, and understanding directions via bus route. However, the clinic staff did not understand the woman's hardship and did not accommodate the patient. Consequently, the highly upset patient sought a local healer instead of pursuing mainstream health care. The patient's complaints of stomach pain were not assessed, nor appropriate diagnostic testing prescribed, resulting in delayed diagnosis of peptic ulcer, which caused internal bleeding.

Leininger's Theoretical Assumption	APN Clinician	APN Leader	APN Educator
Culturally congruent nursing care can only happen when the patient, family, or community values, expressions, or patterns are known and used appropriately, and in meaningful ways by the nurse with the people.	Include lateness as an assessment opportunity to understand cultural value of time and to understand existing SDOH impacts on an individual's pursuit of health care treatment.	Implement staff policies that accommodate for late appointments with a referral to additional services after second late appointment, which addresses potential SDOH impacts.	Offer cultural knowledge workshops to students and staff demonstrating cultural incongruence between patient values and staff/provider expectations.

As the world becomes more interconnected, transcultural nursing will remain an indispensable tool for promoting effective health care delivery and bridging gaps between diverse cultural backgrounds (Sagar & Sagar, 2018). According to Sagar and Sagar (2018), cultural competence is a vital skill that has the power to transform health care delivery by bridging gaps in understanding, communication, and trust. Cultural competence, as it is defined and demonstrated in Leininger's transcultural theory, plays a significant role in reducing health care disparities and improving patient outcomes.

Person and Unmasking Health Disparities: Martinsen's Philosophy of Caring

In the nursing metaparadigm, the essence of the person includes not only being the recipient of care but also encompasses one's spirituality, culture, social network, and socioeconomic status. These integral factors make way for the APN to identify existing and potential health disparities, which may lead to unwanted or poor health outcomes. The core of the person is a focus for the nurse to strive to understand individual needs, preferences, and values to develop patient-centered, holistic care. Without the comprehensive assessment of the person, nursing can neglect identification of health disparities and negative influences creating roadblocks to health and wellness. As a predominant goal in health care is to empower patient self-efficacy in managing one's health, many persons are left to supplement health information, direction of care, and critical understanding of risk factors, leading to negative health outcomes and increasing demands on tertiary care.

Kari Martinsen's (2006) philosophy of caring assumes human beings are social and dependent on other people, called interdependence. As nursing strives to advocate and uphold human dignity, the core role of caring extends beyond the point of care and includes awareness, identification, and action toward ethical practice on a community level. Widespread health disparities heighten the essence of nursing as a vocation committed to moral practice. Martinsen's phenomenological philosophy of caring spotlights nursing as a relationship-based, authentic, and connected practice. A major premise of Martinsen's philosophy calls on nursing to intertwine caring with nursing practice. Under Martinsen's (1991) philosophy of caring, it is critical for nursing to notice the need for care by responding with practical action or an expression of caring. Martinsen (1991) explains the essential element of care is the ability to recognize the need of the other and to act, creating a nursing edict to address the care needs of all.

> *"Care is to be concrete and present in a relationship by our senses and our bodies. It is always to be in a movement away from ourselves and towards the other."*
>
> *—Martinsen (1991, p. 11)*

Martinsen describes care as a trinity: relational, practical, and moral simultaneously practiced. The philosophy supports nursing to extend beyond conventional knowing and doing to connecting with and sustaining others. Martinsen (2006) further offers the concept of dwelling, which is a phenomenological concept related to a sense of belonging, being safe, and feeling at home. Martinsen (2006) posited dwelling is under pressure in modern health care. Under Martinsen's position, client satisfaction is more than following protocols but a deeper connection between humanity. Nursing practice requires skills and education on caring practice, which center around investment of time and applying knowledge of holism rather than approaching clients as a mere extension of their disease when the nurse acts strictly in a utilitarian manner.

With this principal interpretation of caring, APNs can translate caring as a moral attribute recognizing the needs of humans from all socioeconomic levels, linking health disparities to the creation of human need(s). Martinsen calls for nursing to use judgment from a moral framework, which entails widening the view beyond the boundaries of health care culture that are inundated with rules and instead offering moments (time) of mutual respect between nurse and client. This time allows the person to show themselves in the present before being placed in health care's rigid classifications. For the nurse/APN, Martinsen's philosophy creates opportunities through a moral commitment of caring to address health disparities.

Nursing and Unmasking Health Disparities: Boykin and Schoenhofer's Theory of Nursing as Caring

According to the Robert Wood Johnson Foundation (2019), up to 80% of a person's health is determined by socioeconomic factors, health-related behaviors, and environmental conditions. The statistics regarding the effects of SDOH are consistent and emphasize the critical importance for nursing to be present in the efforts to address conditions such as low income, limited education, and geographically tied residences. Due to the negative health outcomes highly associated with SDOH, national medical and nursing associations are calling for the use of social risk screening tools. This is a ground-level approach that is limited in its effectiveness to eliminate potential health risks. Nursing is called to engage in broader innovative approaches to not only incorporate policy- and systems-level changes but to include transforming nursing/caring practice. Returning to nursing theory guides the profession to react in an ontological approach to reach the nature of human need for caring and interconnectedness.

For more information on an example of a social risk screening tool, please review the link to the Centers for Medicare and Medicaid Services developed the Accountable Health Communities (AHC) Health-Related Social Needs (HRSN) screening tool: https://www.cms.gov/priorities/innovation/files/worksheets/ahcm-screeningtool.pdf.

- The Centers for Medicare and Medicaid Services developed the AHC HRSN screening tool to address the critical gap between clinical care and community services.

- This unique 10-question tool assesses five key domains of health-related social needs, collecting a breadth of information that increases the likelihood of identifying significant needs.
- The tool can also be integrated into multiple clinical workflows and is accessible across diverse patient populations.

Critical Reflection: A Kaleidoscope View of SDOH

Aaliyah was 22 years old, homeless, and sleeping outside when she first started coming to an urban (grant-funded) clinic for management of bipolar I disorder. A few weeks after an initial visit, she returned to the clinic pregnant. Aaliyah had run away from an abusive family as an adolescent where her family did not recognize mental illness and spent the last 5 years on the street. Her boyfriend, also a runaway youth with anger management issues and ADHD, came with her to her first prenatal appointment. Neither had any financial resources, no family connections, and no knowledge of the Medicaid system, and they used local shelters, when available, for housing. During her prenatal care, clinic staff and health care providers helped her obtain Medicaid benefits and referred her to a youth counseling program that provided case management and housing. By the time she gave birth, Aaliyah and her boyfriend were living together in a rented room of a house through a voucher program.

After the birth of a healthy, term infant, the family returned to the clinic. The newborn's Medicaid had not been processed, and the couple did not know how to apply for benefits provided by the Special Supplemental Nutrition Program for Women, Infants, and Children (WIC). Aaliyah was breastfeeding but did not own a pump, had only one bottle, and was struggling to keep up her milk supply. She and her boyfriend had no source of income to buy diapers or clothes. Their love for their child was evident, but they were struggling as young new parents who had never witnessed a healthy family environment. The newborn was not gaining weight, and Aaliyah was struggling with depression. Clinic staff focused an increasing amount of time on the family's social condition. With the exception of Aaliyah's bipolar I disorder; the family's health problems fell largely outside of the scope of traditional health care. They needed infant supplies, parenting education, Medicaid, economic resources, food, safe housing, and social support—a sense of dwelling. These social needs stemmed from systemic issues of poverty, family violence, the affordable housing crisis, and historical issues with mental health equality. Postpartum visits and well-child checkups that did not address these underlying issues would do little to improve the health of this family.

Consider the following critical reflections:

- Identify both Aaliyah and her boyfriend's current SDOH.
- Rationalize the link between chronic stress cause by SDOH on Aaliyah's, her newborn's, and her boyfriend's health outcomes.

- Consider an interdisciplinary collaborative approach to addressing SDOH and describe what this might look like for your specific APN role (clinician, leader, educator).
- How would social risk screening at the primary, secondary, and tertiary levels of care make an impact on decreasing health disparities?

Boykin and Schoenhofer's (2013) theory of nursing as caring defines *caring* as the deliberate and embodied realization of value and connectedness. Under the assumptions of the theory, nursing is the only discipline that views providing care as a core value and the explicit goal of its practice (Boykin & Schoenhofer, 2013). The intention of nursing practice is within the context of caring for people directly. Nursing practice is accomplished through purposeful relationships and sincere acts of caring; hence, the theory provides the framework for nursing to fully understand its purpose. Through this implicit understanding, nurses and APNs have presence and resolution to identify health disparities, challenge the causes of SDOH, and advocate for substantial change in health care access and delivery.

TABLE 10.2 Connecting Nursing as Caring to APN Specialty Roles

Basic Premise of Nursing as Caring Theory	APN Clinician	APN Leader	APN Educator
The nurse endeavors to come to know the other as a caring person and seeks to understand how that person might be sustained, supported, and strengthened in their unique process of living caring and growing caring (Boykin & Schoenhofer, 2013).	Enter each patient relationship with recognition of the individual as unique. Demonstrate authentic APN clinician and client encounters with active listening and respond to needs accordingly.	Integrate assessment of caring and provide caring orientation to the screening of entry-level nursing positions.	Incorporate self-awareness as a skill in nursing education with the purpose of empowering nurses to take responsibility of their practice by seeking and applying knowledge.

Environment and Unmasking Health Disparities: Roger's Theory of Unitary Human Beings

In the nursing metaparadigm, the environment includes the physical environment and social factors that influence a person's health. To stay within these contexts would limit the nurse's practice of caring. An advanced view of the environment includes not only health (outcomes) but cultural, political, and economic factors. It is within this very domain of the metaparadigm that nursing can address health disparities as a natural association to its practice of caring for the purpose of nurses is to promote wellbecoming for all persons and environments (Malinski, 2022).

Within the theoretical framework of Martha Roger's theory of unitary human beings, the person (unitary human being) and their environment are one. A basic assumption of Roger's theory states a person cannot be separated from their environment when attending to health. Roger provides nursing with a clear delineation of a person under the defining elements of unitary beings. According to Rogers (1970), persons are not separate entities but integrated beings whose experiences cannot be reduced to individual parts. A distinct concept in Roger's theory is *openness* in that people interact with their environment with meaning. Openness is a characteristic of energy fields, which Roger (1970) defines as the fundamental unit of the living and the nonliving, whereas persons and the environment are energy fields or have a dynamic (fluid) relationship with one another. Roger's collective attributes to describe a human being say that nursing can deduce the undeniable influence a person and their environment can have on one another. Roger's theory sheds light on the interconnectivity of a person and their environment as unified and without boundaries. With this openness, the APN can address health disparities by understanding the process of co-evolution. The person and their environment cannot adapt or find equilibrium when both systems are dynamic and ever-changing. Rather, negentropy exists within living systems, moving toward diversity, innovation, creativity, and complexity (Rogers, 1970). In addressing health disparities, Roger's theory offers the nurse and APN an understanding of the dynamic relationship between person and the environment. Because the environment has many factors (social, cultural, physical, and political), the APN can apply Roger's theory as a philosophical approach to providing a path toward health, wellness, and openness.

Figure Credit

Fig. 10.1: The National Academies of Sciences, Engineering, and Medicine, "Areas of Activity to Strengthen Integration of Social Care into Health Care," Integrating Social Care into the Delivery of Health Care: Moving Upstream to Improve the Nation's Health. Copyright © 2019 by National Academies Press.

CHAPTER 11

Aligning Theory to Ethical Challenges

Key Terms

Ethics: The art of assuming responsibility for others, for humanity, for the Earth, and of self-questioning (Bommier, 2019).

Organizational ethics: The applied ethics discipline that addresses the moral choices influenced and guided by values, standards, principles, rules, and strategies associated with organizational activities and business situations (Letendre, 2015).

Self-actualization: Everything you are capable of becoming (Maslow, 1965).

Introduction

There is little doubt the pandemic impacted health care professionals and staffs' physical, social, and mental well-being and their ability to remain resilient. The pandemic commanded the rapid development and accelerated deployment of new technologies integrating AI components. In reflection of COVID-19 and its direct challenges placed on the U.S. health care system, most health care professionals can attest to challenges related to fair and equitable allocation of scarce resources. Despite the magnification of these issues, they are not new to the health care system nationwide. Nurses were faced with countless ethical challenges, both for themselves and their patients, which often left many feeling defeated and without support.

Technology was an instant resource during the pandemic to create a sense of belonging and connections. Big data and machine learning have an impact on most aspects of modern life and have been for quite some time. The optimism of AI applications in health care has persisted with the hopes it can substantially improve all areas of health care, from diagnostics to treatment (Bohr & Memarzadeh, 2020). Administrative workflow, clinical documentation, and patient outreach are being utilized with AI features such as enhanced patient monitoring (Bohr & Memarzadeh, 2020). With the increasing demand for health care services and the shortage of health care providers, technology has been utilized as a steady route to find real-time solutions. Despite the expanding health care infrastructure being guided by AI, perpetuation of ethical comportment for the APN remains a priority concern as many technology applications are generally linked to less personalized patient care and limiting the time of the care provider to ensure trust and authenticity in provider–patient relationships.

Ethics is one of the vital components of health and medical care in general, and in the public health care sector in special (Kooli, 2021). Name a few ethical challenges would potentially minimize the overall need for ethical care to be heightened as a top priority. For context, the following challenges are presented for the APN to consider in preparation of their new role and scope of practice. According to Buntin (2021), major challenges are related to health insurance coverage, the solvency of publicly funded programs, the stability of the health care safety net, market power and consolidation, inequities in health care access and outcomes, public health infrastructure, and the failure to effectively use technology to help counteract these problems. As health care costs skyrocket ($4 trillion in 2020, or an estimated 18% of GDP), and health care systems continue to be consolidated, incomplete insurance coverage for many people is a tangible consequence that creates higher premium prices (Centers for Medicare & Medicaid Services, n.d.). Combine the unaffordability of health care coverage and the growing number of vulnerable populations and more citizens face more widespread reduced access to essential care services. As a result, the APN is confronted with balancing quality care with efficiency, being advocates for increased access to affordable care, supporting a strong health care workforce (mentoring colleagues), ensuring clear communication to assist others in informed decision-making, and becoming participatory in health care research, leadership, and the education of the future health care workforce.

One proposed solution is to change the way ethics is encountered in health care. Traditional health care ethics is focused on the individual, whereas health care within "organizational ethics" focuses on collectives, which include groups of clinicians, patients, nonclinical workers, administrators, and the institution (Phelan, 2020). The response to ethical challenges is an understanding for the need for change. Change at the organizational level will employ a broader and universal response that addresses more than just structure but also the culture in which health care is offered and delivered. The APN clinician, leader, and educator are purveyors of ethical care and simultaneously advocates for change. Nursing theory offers the APN a framework to directly address ethical issues within the nursing metaparadigm.

This chapter will explore the following learning objectives in relation to poor patient outcomes:

1. Explore the nursing metaparadigm through the challenges set forth post-pandemic related to ethical issues and considerations for the APN in practice.
2. Align selected nursing theories and models to each domain of the nursing metaparadigm: health, person, nurse, and environment.
3. Analyze the role of APN clinician, leader, and educator to address ethical challenges to apply clinical specialty skills through the guidance of nursing theory to assist patient pursuits to health and wellness.

Nursing Metaparadigm: Addressing Ethical Challenges

Ethics is an inherent and inseparable part of health care, whereas the health care provider has an ethical obligation to benefit the patient, to avoid or minimize harm, and to respect the values and preferences of the patient (Varkey, 2020a). Four major ethical principles are embedded in the education, licensure, and daily practice of the APN: autonomy, nonmaleficence, beneficence, and justice. Each of the four principles call for the APN to recognize their existence in all health care encounters and sponsor change when inequities are present. The APN is driven by personal ethics, disciplinary regulation, and professional guidance to view ethical challenges through the lens of the metaparadigm. Just as technology has offered new ways to enhance workflow and gather/monitor data, the APN is a beacon of advocacy for the person on the receiving end of health care, whether the person is actively seeking care or is trapped without access. Viewing ethical issues through both the lens of the APN and the person creates a continuum of just care, which creates synergy and a healthy environment for both to flourish.

Health and Ethical Challenges: Newman's Health as Expanding Consciousness

COVID-19 impacted the mistrust many patients felt towards health care systems, particularly when there were missed or unclear public communications regarding the rationales (evidence) behind public health mandates. Accountability has become a highly regarded criterion for the public to seek and receive health care services. Notwithstanding the fear borne from COVID, health continues to be a universal ambition persons pursue with or without the support of institutional health care services. As ethical concerns continue to grow and be masked by multiple barriers, such as coverage inefficiencies and poor (population) representation, APNs are a bridge between health and illness, just policies, and competent education.

Critical Reflection

With the expanding demands on health care and providers, do you see ethics as a separate specialty that can be integrated into the framework of health care?

Margaret Newman enriched the profession and practice of nursing by presenting a fresh, holistic vision of the person seeking health (care). Newman's vision recognized evolving patterns. By incorporating Newman's (1994) transformative paradigm of nursing as "caring in the health experience," the APN recognizes patterns as changing through good health and chaos (disease). By describing health as patterns of disease and the evolution of the unitary pattern of the whole person, Newman laid forth a nursing practice principle that permitted both the nurse and the patient to partner in recognizing these patterns. By virtue of ethical practice (care), the APN also recognizes the environment as being influential on one's health and often contributes greatly to its chaos, or disease origins and exacerbations. Since the nurse often enters the patient's experience during times of chaos, the nurse is integral in providing action, which upholds ethical standards of care.

> *If the future of nursing is to be strong and of greatest service to the health of the global community, nursing practice must be deeply rooted in the knowledge of the discipline while responding with agility to societal trends and conditions.*
> *—Pharris (2011, p. 193)*

Through Newman's theory of health as expanding consciousness, the APN can view a patient's patterns of behavior, and when assessed holistically the APN, in return, offers no judgment and becomes authentically present. Authentic presence provides opportunities to engage in meaningful communication while potentially disclosing influences or societal values the patient holds that may be impacting their health goals. The application of Newman's theory offers the APN a view of the patient that is not defined by disease, condition, or illness, but rather as an interaction with the person as a unified whole.

For the APN, exploring Newman's theory promotes self-actualization for both the provider and the patient. Self-actualization, according to Abraham Maslow (1965), is everything you are capable of becoming. An essential characteristic of self-actualization is understanding it is unique to the individual. Self-actualization reveals a deeply embedded characteristic of nurses demonstrating autonomy and objective concern about humanity. Understanding and being a steward of Newman's (1994) theory enables the APN to see beyond self to ethically practice nursing care with continuous observations of patterns, meaning, and holism, in other words "caring in the health experience."

Person and Ethical Challenges: Barker's Tidal Model of Mental Health Recovery

Persons are unique in every dimension: physical, emotional, social, and spiritual. Individual responses to disease, crises, and health challenges are met with a choice of reactive behaviors that may or may not lead to healthy outcomes. Since COVID-19's outbreak, people have had a wide range of responses to a potential deadly communicable disease. For some, the response has been positive, such as becoming more present with their daily health choices (behavior), while others have had a difficult transition from lockdown to living in a world where COVID exists. The impact to people's psyche has been widespread, creating challenges beyond life before the disease, and many of these challenges have been met with increasing ethical conflicts.

Mental health issues, such as substance use disorders, anxiety, sleep disorders, depression, suicides, posttraumatic stress disorders, and panic disorders, have risen significantly since the onset of COVID and have impacted vulnerable populations at an even higher rate (Vadivel et al., 2021). Not only has there been new onset of mental health conditions but also a relapse of preexisting mental illness. Mental health services were overloaded after the lockdowns and had minimal preparation to support these needed services and mental health providers. A cycle of fear persisted for many people experiencing financial insecurity, creating barriers to accessing mental health care. According to Vijayaraghavan et al. (2011), a substantial body of evidence suggests that people with the highest level of mental health needs often have the least access to services. In a post-COVID-19 pandemic era, it is exaggerated, owing to an economic recession, strain on resources, and unemployment (Vadivel et al., 2021). The APN has an ethical duty to address mental health in all patients.

By knowing a person as an entity of evolving dimensions, the APN takes an active role in identification and intervention to assist in mental health/recovery. According to Ransing et al. (2020), interventions are needed to reduce stigmatization and discrimination toward minority or vulnerable groups and to inform policy changes. General and specific interventions should be directed toward identification of drivers (e.g., misinformation), facilitators (e.g., lack of regulations), and intersecting factors (e.g., occupation, such as health care workers) toward reducing stigma and discrimination (Ransing et al., 2020). An active process of outreach by the APN, in any role, clinician, leader, or educator, can make a significant impact on supporting persons' mental health goals, hence demonstrating ethical care.

Barker's (1996) tidal model of mental health recovery helps nurses comprehend the meaning of mental health from the patient's point of view, as well as how the patient can be helped to start or be supported on a journey of recovery. According to Barker (1996), the starting point of this theory is immediate care, what the patient is experiencing at that moment and what should be done to overcome the crisis at hand. APNs are encouraged and supported through Barker's theory to address mental health needs following a philosophy that integrates individualized holistic care. The model provides a structure for all APNs despite their specialty practice to connect with the patient at the place the patient presents physically, mentally, and spiritually. Barker provides a visual representation of a well-formed process the APN, in all care settings, can use to address mental health needs based on three phases (see Figure 11.1). As a continuum model, Barker provides the APN with the concept of developmental care, which focuses on long-term support and is centered on the patient as the driver (owner) of their recovery. As Figure 11.1 illustrates, a crisis is met with focused care and short-term solution(s), but as the patient is supported through the next two phases, an ownership evolves, and a deeper understanding of mental health needs/illness is explored. The APN managing ethical conflicts in real time faces similar context: As the ethical dilemma is initially met, the APN uses previous experiential knowledge and commitment to nursing ethical standards, but as transitions occur over time, they can probe into cause-and-effect factors to permit extended reflection and peer discussions to address similar ethical issues.

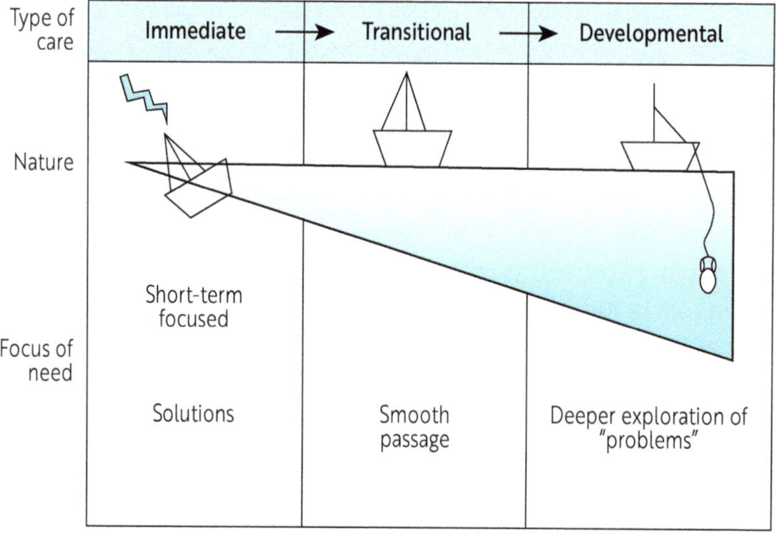

FIGURE 11.1 The tidal model care continuum.

A description of the person is provided in a highly outlined perspective to assist the APN in their specific roles. *Person* is defined by Barker (2003) in three domains: self, world, and others. APNs can specialize care through each distinct role of clinician, leader, and educator based on these domains while upholding an ethical standard to support mental health.

TABLE 11.1 APN Clinician, Leader, and Educator: Addressing Mental Health Through the Lens of Barker's Definition of *Person*

Domains of 'Person" (Barker, 2003)	APN Clinician	APN Leader	APN Educator
Self	Recognize a patient's fears and where the patient presents in the moment.	Identify staff and other providers' beliefs of mental health care, with acknowledgement of these beliefs in daily decisions to support the unit/system's work productivity.	Create a curriculum that promotes acknowledgement of student feelings and functions through a philosophy of "learning through caring."
World	Demonstrate understanding of the patient's life experiences as part of their mental health outcomes.	Establish and cultivate a work culture/environment that welcomes the sharing of beliefs and individual thoughts to support collective decision-making.	Promote student-centered curriculum, with recognition of student achievements and further educational needs.
Others	Include family, social support persons specific to the patient when addressing mental health needs.	Ensure a team approach to pol icy decision and change.	Initiate a peer community of learners to support one another.

Mental well-being is a standard of ethical care. APNs can lead in mental health care by viewing nursing theory through a systematic and creative lens. Nursing theory as a practical tool creates a supportive framework that embraces the unique roles of the APN and the unique needs of the person.

Nursing and Ethical Challenges: Watson's Self-Care Theory

Nursing continues to be voted as one of the most ethical and honest professions (Saad, 2023). Nursing, despite its deep dedication to holistic practice in that every person is respected with dignity and integrity, experiences barriers to their ethical philosophy of care due to time constraints, burnout, and blurred lines of ethical decision-making. Findings from the ANA (2017) health risk appraisal revealed that 68% of surveyed nurses put their patients' health, safety, and wellness before their own. Nurses and APNs persistently make moral decisions in their respective roles by weighing consequences and aiming to do good; however, studies show that a lack of congruence between the practice and ideals of care causes ethical dilemmas for nurses (Haahr et al., 2019). Holm et al. (2013) highlight that ethical dilemmas arise from conflicts among values, norms, and interests, which can be understood as the tension of knowing the "right thing to do but experiencing institutional or other constraints making it difficult to pursue the desired course of action" (p. 403). As a result, many nurses and APNs experience threats to their own health. According to Linton and Koonmen (2020), PTSD, burnout, moral distress, compassion fatigue, and suicide are becoming more prevalent in the nursing profession. Nurses give the best care to patients when they are operating at the peak of their own wellness (Linton & Koonmen, 2020). To achieve optimal practice performance, self-care can be an effective tool, yet many nurses and APNs hold a misconception of self-care as indulgent.

> *"Embracing a care-based perspective recognizes that nurses live in a web of moral duties that includes their duty to protect themselves, their patients, their families, and communities."*
>
> *—AACN (2017, para 2)*

The APN enters a scope of practice that can profoundly impact how ethical decisions are made by safeguarding their autonomy and commitment to just care. APNs must be reminded of the ANA code of ethics, which explicitly states nurses must adopt self-care as a duty to self in addition to their duty to care for patient. To champion the nurse and APN in meeting these ethical challenges in day-to-day practice, Jean Watson's self-care theory can provide a framework to address the support required so that nurses and APNs can practice to the fullest of their skills, knowledge, and scope.

> *"We have to learn how to offer caring, love, forgiveness, compassion, and mercy to ourselves before we can offer authentic caring and love to others."*
>
> *—Linton and Koonmen (2020, p. 1694)*

Watson's "caring science" is an evolving philosophical, ethical, and epistemic field of study grounded in nursing (Watson Caring Science Institute, 2023). According to Watson (2008), a nurse/APN cannot practice within the professional caring-healing model without learning how to love and care for self. Watson's theory posits a foundation for fostering nurse well-being and attainment of self-actualization. As discussed previously, self-actualization opens opportunities for full realization of one's ability to reach satisfaction in their being and professional lives. The process of self-care through the framework of Watson is not simple or even comfortable at times, but it is through this important work nurse/APNs can practice to the fullest extent of their role while fulfilling a duty to self.

Environment and Ethical Challenges: Roy's Adaptation of Nursing Model

Today's health care environment has persistent ethical challenges, creating the need for APNs to be versatile in practice to maintain moral strength and creating a dichotomy of care. Balancing efficiency in practice while promoting health for all is a complex and ever-changing skill set. Without the continual presence of ethical comportment, health care and their providers risk losing patient trust and potentially those who may neglect their own health necessities. A major complex ethical issue regarding the environment rests in the question of how APNs can impact and call for change. As many people are influenced by the environment in which they live, statistics, such as that 6 million people die from hunger or malnutrition and tens of thousands of people die to risks associated with homelessness, will remain part of the social fabric of many communities (The Hastings Center, 2023). How can the APN address the multitude of environmental influences, which often carry ethical issues? The answer may be found in understanding and applying the concept of adaptation.

Roy (1997) defined *adaptation* as the process and outcome by which the thinking and feeling person uses conscious awareness and choice to create human and environmental integrations. The APN can look to Roy's adaptation of nursing model to understand the interrelationships between the person, health, and the environment. Just as the nursing metaparadigm addresses each domain (including the nurse), Roy's theory of adaptation offers a clear pathway for the APN to integrate its theoretical assumptions to everyday practice.

Roy describes the environment as stimuli that impacts behavior and the ability to adapt (Roy et al., 2009). According to Roy (1997), one's health continuum is shaped by responses of environmental stimuli. When an individual experiences a stimulus or a change in their environment, stress is present. Stress is the body's response to a change requiring adaptation (healthy or unhealthy). This is true for both the APN and the patient. Just as Roy's theory can be applied to the patient's needs, adaptation is a critical and essential skill for the APN to sustain ethical care. As the APN recognizes health as a state of being and becoming whole, the APN can apply this principle to addressing ethical dilemmas in their environment. The environment is a powerful stimuli for people's choices, often leading to ethical considerations for the APN in practice. Roy's (1997) description of environmental stimuli as focal (internal or external), contextual, or residual can be utilized as a framework for the APN to address root causes (influences) of ethical dilemmas.

TABLE 11.2 APN Clinician, Leader, and Educator: Exploring Roy's Environmental Stimuli to Address Ethical Challenges and Support an Adaptive Response

Environmental Stimuli (Roy, 1997)	APN Clinician	APN Leader	APN Educator
Focal (Internal and External)	Enhance evaluation methods to detect stimuli that present major concern(s) for the patient at the moment/time they are seeking care.	Enhance evaluation of staff–staff, staff–patient, and staff–public interactions.	Enhance evaluation of student learning.
Response/ Adaptation	Employ a holistic assessment process (skill) that identifies immediate (focal) impetuses affecting health outcomes.	Employ a nonbiased assessment of staff productivity and work culture.	Employ a continuous formative process to determine successful student outcomes.
Contextual	Gain knowledge of patient population characteristics, including cultural values/ beliefs and the environments in which they live, work, and socially interact.	Gain knowledge of workplace culture and vision/mission of the institution in which health care is provided.	Gain knowledge of student population characteristics, including cultural values/ beliefs and the environments in which they live, work, and socially interact.
Response/ Adaptation	Be present and actively assess for immediate stimuli affecting the patient's health and reason(s) for seeking health care.	Engage with staff on a consistent level, which promotes understanding of current workplace issues while incorporating a team-centric approach to policy development.	Build and adjust curriculum that supports various learning styles and needs.

TABLE 11.2 APN Clinician, Leader, and Educator: Exploring Roy's Environmental Stimuli to Address Ethical Challenges and Support an Adaptive Response (*Continued*)

Environmental Stimuli (Roy, 1997)	APN Clinician	APN Leader	APN Educator
Residual	Be aware of unseen factors challenging one's ability to choose healthy behaviors.	Be aware of unseen factors challenging staff ability to effectively meet employee/role expectations and responsibilities.	Be aware of unseen factors challenging students and educators to effectively learn and instruct.
Response/ Adaptation	Broaden perspectives through a biopsychosocial lens that captures unknown controls of one's ability to reach health goals.	Broaden perspectives through a biopsychosocial lens that captures unknown controls of one's ability to reach job satisfaction and productivity.	Broaden perspectives through a biopsychosocial lens that captures unknown controls of one's ability to reach educational and professional goals.

Ethical challenges are a mainstay in both the health care and educational environments. Barriers to good health and quality education are ethical dilemmas requiring attention of the APN. Through the innovative use of nursing theory, APNs can address, change, and secure the practice of ethical care/standards. The road will never be easy, but a commitment to moral courage and resilience will create change.

Figure Credit

Fig. 11.1: P.J. Barker and P. Buchanan-Barker, "The Tidal Model Care Continuum," The Tidal Model: A Guide for Mental Health Professionals, p. 42. Copyright © 2005 by Taylor & Francis Group.

PART IV

Refreshing Theory as a Practical Tool for the APN

Locally, by state, nation, and on a global level, health care is challenged daily, from overworked staff, increasing chronic care complexities, technology adaptations, skyrocketing costs, and limited supplies. APNs have been answering the calls of health care systems while expanding their roles to meet these challenges with skill and a commitment to caring. The COVID-19 pandemic created a major burden on what was an already struggling health care system to provide quality care for many. These post-pandemic challenges have been summarized and reviewed through the lens of the nursing metaparadigm, with an application of nursing theory, to offer prospects for the APN to be creative yet grounded in nursing's core values.

Five Prevailing Post-Pandemic Health Care/ Educational Challenges Explored

- Remote care/education
- Health care costs/education costs
- Poor patient outcomes/student outcomes
- Health care disparities/educational disparities
- Ethical challenges
    - Nurse's safety
    - Patient/student safety

- Role and moral distress
- Resource allocation
- APN clinician–patient relationship
- APN leader–staff relationship
- APN educator–student relationship

In the health care system, no one more than the nurse felt the weighted impact of the pandemic on both professional and personal levels. Nursing's core values were tested, much like those of our nursing predecessors in times of war. Nursing prevailed, and through the long, often dismal tunnel of COVID, nursing persisted and continued to further its professional role into advanced nursing practice. Now is a time for hope and a remembrance of struggles that created many learning moments. As nurses remain the most trusted profession post-pandemic (Aiken et al., 2021), the realization of an opportunity to grow and make change to a debilitated health care system is upon the profession. Through experience, reflection, and continued growth, the APN can look forward to a brighter future in which their unique role can make strong influences on health care delivery, leadership, and education. Since the pandemic, a unique time exists for the nurse and the APN to identify the changes to care expectations and to create opportunities to innovate caring practices, influence policy and decisions regarding health care organization, adapt education to meet the health care environment's skill needs, and work collaboratively with interdisciplinary teams through the guidance and support of nursing theory.

The APN is in an exceptional position to reevaluate the usability of nursing theory.

CHAPTER 12

MetaPORT

An Algorithm for the APN to Apply Theory to Practice

Key Terms

Cognitive restructuring: A therapeutic process that helps the client discover, challenge, and modify or replace their negative, irrational thoughts (Clark, 2013).

Community of practice (CoP): An APN-led group of health care colleagues, both nursing and interdisciplinary, who share ideas and perceptions related to health care issues.

Executive function: The set of neurocognitive processes that help with impulse control, attention, working memory, and cognitive flexibility (Stucke, 2021).

Root-cause analysis: The process of discovering the root causes of problems to systematically prevent and solve underlying issues rather than just treating ad hoc symptoms (Tableau, n.d.).

SWOT analysis: A situational analysis carried out for different purposes (Contributor, 2021).

Introduction

According to the International Council of Nurses (ICN, 2020), the APN has an expert knowledge base that integrates research, education, care practice, and management in a highly autonomous role. The APN is prepared to be an autonomous provider, leader, and educator, yet these roles are met with demands that can stagnate their progress toward making a positive impact. Ensuring time for reflection is critical for the APN. Through reflection, the APN can create synergy between past learning and future innovation. Advancing the role of the nurse and APN comes with a commitment to core professional values and an understanding of how care practices can adapt to the environment without compromising a dutiful, holistic approach. To strengthen the foundation of nursing practice, the APN can look to nursing theory as a grounded framework to not only remain true to nursing ethics but to also guide advanced nursing practice. Nursing theory is foundational to how the nursing profession is defined and is recommended to be reunderstood as a practical tool rather than an abstract concept linked to the nursing metaparadigm. A pragmatic algorithm titled MetaPORT is proposed to assist the APN to reflect and apply nursing theory within their unique environments. Each essential step of the algorithm will be presented to create a process of critical thinking for the APN to use nursing theory as a tool to address their unique practice challenges.

This chapter will explore the following learning objectives in relation to practical application of nursing theory:

1. Present the MetaPORT algorithm as a practical tool to use nursing theory as a guide to create synergy and innovation in the APNs unique roles.
2. Define each step of the MetaPORT process.

MetaPORT Key

SWOT: Strengths, weakness, opportunities, and threats
RCA: Root-cause analysis
NT: Nursing theory
CoP: Community of practice

Meta *(Metacognition)*	**PORT**
Calm the mind **U**se reflection **E**valuate (Apply SWOT analysis)	**P**roblem identification • Review literature and apply RCA **O**rganize thinking • Create a thinking diary **R**elationship to NT • Compare/contrast issue with NT assumptions **T**alk out loud • Adopt a CoP

FIGURE 12.1 MetaPORT diagram.

MetaPORT: Metacognition

Metacognition is an effort to enhance well-being through cognitive and emotional domains. When beginning the process of MetaPORT, the APN will apply the acronym CUE (calming the mind, using reflection, and evaluation). CUE initiates the intentional work of the APN to examine the issue from past, current, and future lenses. CUE starts with calming the mind. As busy health care professionals, time is elusive, and often APNs handle multiple issues simultaneously. Thinking on your feet becomes second nature and often dominates intentional thought processes. Training the mind to think with clarity provides the APN with mental regulation or opens the thought pathways to distinctively think about a specific issue/concern. In doing so, the issue or concern receives attention in that systematic thought can be applied, opening the intellectual doorway to solutions.

There are multiple ways to clear the mind, from meditation to journaling. One method that may prove to be effective for the APN is to employ cognitive restructuring. Cognitive restructuring is a therapeutic technique to notice and change negative or unproductive thinking patterns. When juggling multiple issues that require answers and direction, emotional responses may take precedence, which restricts positive and efficient thinking patterns while inhibiting innovation. The APN, in any setting, manages multiple judgment-based decisions that may lack a clear, definitive answer, particularly when considering the barriers seen in today's health care environment. Some ways to engage in cognitive restructuring include self-monitoring and questioning assumptions. Self-monitoring requires attention to one's thinking and recognizing when negative feelings become present. Actively disengaging in these moments can clear the mind for more productive thought. Questioning assumptions enables analysis of what one's thoughts are based on, such as emotion or even inaccurate information. Through both methods, the APN can quickly learn how they respond to thinking during stressful situations while determining factors that may influence either a positive or negative (catastrophic) thinking approach. In these moments, the APN can learn to think in a free-flowing, nonjudgmental, and positive manner.

The next phase of metacognition is to use reflection. It is important to note the process of reflection has an incredible personal effect, and this is the enhancement of self-concept. When one believes they can achieve a goal, the process becomes more vibrant. Not only is the APN engaged in critical thinking to practice safely and more effectively, but the APN also simultaneously engages in personal growth. The act of metacognition provides the APN a starting point to think without distraction and judgment. By placing oneself in a state of metacognition, the APN takes control of their thought processes to connect experiences to knowledge, allowing for more flexible thinking, or executive functioning. Executive functioning is self-regulatory actions to manage time, plan, focus attention, and handle multiple tasks to achieve a goal. To successfully put metacognition and executive functioning to work, reflection is needed. Reflection can be performed as a four-step process:

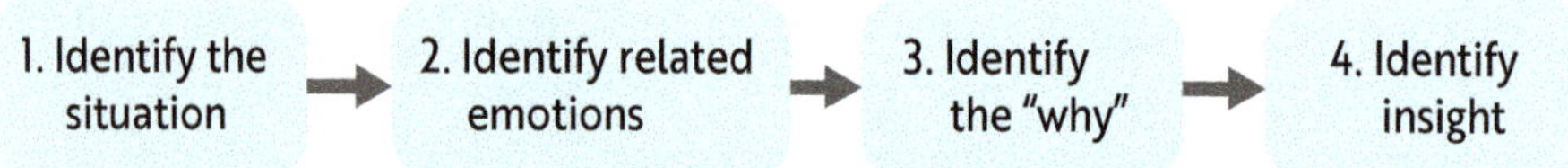

FIGURE 12.2 Four steps to reflection for the APN.

Step 1: Identify the situation. The APN examines two questions: what and who. This is an opportunity to think about the situation in detail, when removed from the moment, for clarity. Consider identifying the situation (or issue) with less thinking noise. Distractions can mask what is truly being observed. Answer who is involved or impacted by the situation.

Step 2: Identify related emotions. The APN has permission to explore how the situation is causing them to feel and be honest about these feelings. Feelings/emotions are powerful, and when used in reflective processes can assist in recognizing similar situations in the future.

Step 3: Identify the why. The APN is afforded the time to recognize unseen details that may have a direct impact on the situation. Through this recognition, the APN may develop enriched perceptions related to solutions.

Step 4: Identify insight. The APN analyzes the situation based on the question "Could I have done something different in the moment?" This can be recognized as permission in that the APN allows themselves the needed time to analyze the situation further to explore positive solutions.

Once reflection is complete, the APN can further the metacognitive process by engaging in evaluation. This is a two-prong approach through evaluation of self and/or the situation. A common evaluation process is the SWOT analysis, which requires the use of humility and unbiased responses to deliver a four-point perspective (see Tables 12.1 and 12.2).

TABLE 12.1 Individual SWOT Analysis

SWOT	Questions to Ask	Response(s)
Strengths	• What personal characteristics align well to my current nursing role? • What have I achieved in my current nursing role?	

TABLE 12.1 Individual SWOT Analysis (*Continued*)

SWOT	Questions to Ask	Response(s)
Weaknesses	• Are there areas of education or training which would provide enhanced understanding of how to manage work-related issues? • Do I avoid certain situations because I lack skills and/or confidence?	
Opportunities	• Am I familiar with opportunities available for professional development at my current place of employment? • Do I understand the mission and values set forth by the environment in which I work?	
Threats	• Do my personal habits (e.g., procrastination) interfere with my ability to perform my nursing role to the fullest of my ability and scope of practice?	

TABLE 12.2 Situational SWOT Analysis

SWOT	Questions to Ask	Response(s)
Strengths	• What characteristics of the situational environment supports a positive and holistic response?	
Weaknesses	• What characteristics of the situational environment do not support a positive and holistic approach?	
Opportunities	• Does the situational environment support innovative thinking? • Does the situation (issue) align to a theoretical framework?	
Threats	• Does the situational environment support the change process?	

Application of metacognition through CUE helps the APN to be openly engaged to become a convergent thinker and change agent. The next step of the MetaPORT algorithm is problem identification.

To learn more about metacognition research, check out the following article:

Fleur, D. S., Bredeweg, B., & Van Den Bos, W. (2021). Metacognition: Ideas and insights from neuro- and educational sciences. *NPJ: Science of Learning*, *6*(1). https://doi.org/10.1038/s41539-021-00089-5

Problem Identification

Throughout the evolution of the role of the nurse, the primary goal steadily remains with patient advocacy and providing safe, quality care on the basis of evidence obtained through research. Problem identification is a critical step and one that does not present itself without metacognitive efforts. Often, situations are embedded into daily practice and professional interactions, resulting in misplaced authenticity of the concern or issue and its implications to the clinician, leader, educator, patient, staff, and student. Post metacognition, the means of identifying the situation/problem is weighted on the efforts of the APN to perform due diligence regarding assessment of current EBP. An issue, concern, or concept related to nursing is not without connections to research. A review of literature answers the question what is the state of the evidence of the selected topic? (Boren & Moxley, 2015). To properly identify the problem, the APN needs to engage in an integrative review of literature.

An integrative review of literature is done for different reasons. For the purpose of applying nursing theory to practice, the goal is to evaluate current practices, create synergy between knowledge and experience, and possibly identify the need for further nursing research. Using an integrative approach to review literature allows for analysis of qualitative and quantitative research through diverse sources, providing the APN with a comprehensive understanding to inform EBP in health care. To expansively understand a problem/issue, APNs can use tools such as a RCA to unveil further insights into reciprocal effects stemming from the issue. As the APN gains more knowledge of factors contributing to the problem, solutions and innovative thinking become part of the MetaPORT process.

TABLE 12.3 An APN Integrative Review of Literature Template

Steps	APN Integrative Review Process Steps	Additional Insights	APN Notes
1	Select topics/concepts aligned to an issue.	Use the reflection and SWOT analysis outcomes to determine topics/issues.	
2	Determine the intent of the review.	Develop a guiding question that is both broad and directs the review toward a purpose.	
3	Perform a literature search.	Use multiple search engines to include both experimental and nonexperimental studies.	
4	Use a data collection table.	Create a data collection tool that represents a two-point scale in that findings are rated as high or low based on quality, rigor (research design), and relevance to research questions (Conn et al., 2003).	

TABLE 12.3 An APN Integrative Review of Literature Template (*Continued*)

Steps	APN Integrative Review Process Steps	Additional Insights	APN Notes
5	Evaluate literature findings.	Using the data collection table, evaluate findings, patterns, emerging themes, and relationships between data sources.	
6	Formulate conclusions.	Summarize findings with a focus on the selected issue/topic.	
7	Apply findings to an RCA.	Conduct an RCA.	

TABLE 12.4 Integrated Review Data Collection Table Template

Source/APA reference citation	Quality	Rigor	Relevance to Research Question	Patterns/ Themes	Relationships Among Data Sources/ Linked to Source #
Source 1 Min, D., Lee, J., & Ahn, J. (2023). A qualitative study on the self-care experiences of people with heart failure. *Western Journal of Nursing Research*, 45(7), 646–652. https://doi.org/10.1177/01939459231169102	Potential bias Small number of participants Low	Qualitative, descriptive, exploratory study using semi-structured interviews High	Aimed to evaluate self-care of patients with heart failure based on their experiences and emotions High	Identify by the findings of the study	Found by reexamining each article's patterns/ themes

In gathering a thorough understanding and identification of a problem (issue), the APN is able to view potential and real-time domino effects from an issue. An RCA is an approach to uncover causes of a problem and to begin steps toward problem solving through evidenced-based solutions. The Joint Commission requires health care institutions to have a comprehensive process in place to analyze sentinel events. An RCA is one of the most commonly used error-analysis tools to lessen adverse events and optimize patient safety by using an investigative analysis process to identify vulnerabilities that can be eliminated or mitigated without focusing on individual reviews. Studies have shown RCA tools often result in ineffective, weak, and unsustainable solutions (Kellogg et al., 2016). Despite RCA's lack of systems-based effectiveness, the APN can use this tool as part of the MetaPORT process to systematically direct specialized nursing practice in a theory-driven and evidence-based methodology. RCAs can be accomplished in different methods, such as a process map or a fishbone diagram. A process map uses a flow chart, and a fishbone diagram uses a visual diagram to capture causes from multiple sources. A fishbone diagram offers a means to brainstorming and mind mapping while being easy to use. Causes discovered from the RCA methods can later be reexamined for renewed approaches to applying solutions or rethinking processes.

RCA Methods

For more information on process (flow) maps to perform an RCA, please see the following link:

- https://www.patientsafety.va.gov/docs/RCA-Guidebook_02052021.pdf

For more information on fishbone diagrams to perform an RCA, please see the following link:

- https://www.cms.gov/Medicare/Provider-Enrollment-and-Certification/QAPI/Downloads/FishboneRevised.pdf

Example Fishbone Diagram for the APN Clinician

Clinical Scenario

A family nurse practitioner (FNP) was caring for an elderly patient in a skilled unit after receiving the resident as an admission 2 days prior. The resident is 72 years old with a history of type II diabetes, hyperthyroidism, GERD, hypertension, depression, and schizoaffective disorder. The resident began to acutely change, exhibiting fever, increased respiratory rate, and complaints of severe abdominal pain. The FNP began a differential diagnostic evaluation, including blood and urine cultures, and while cultures were pending the resident was placed on prophylactic antibiotics; there were no signs of site infection. Both tests were negative, but the resident began to further decline with tachycardia, persistent fever, and lower blood pressure, which required supplemental oxygen. The FNP ordered the resident to be sent to the local emergency department for tertiary diagnostic work-up and supportive care.

The resident was admitted to the ICU with a diagnosis of respiratory failure and septicemia. The FNP continued to follow up with the resident's care in the hospital with the determination to discover the cause for decline and source of sepsis. As the FNP proceeds with the MetaPORT algorithm, a fishbone diagram was used for further resident evaluation.

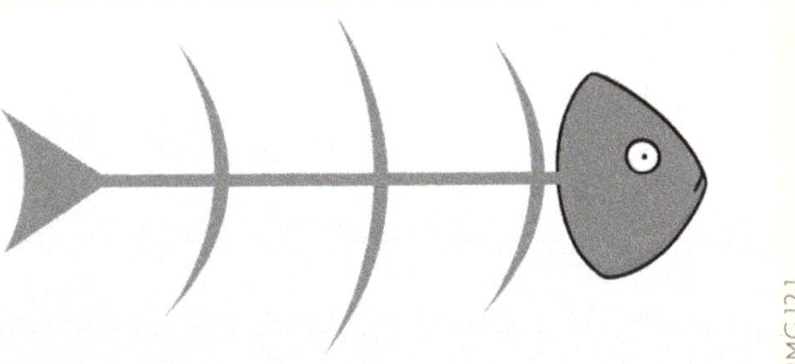

IMG 12.1

Each bone of the diagram was used as a broad category to assist he FNP in evaluating the cause for the resident's acute decline and need for further tertiary care. For example, the broad categories can include full review of medications, sources of infection, environment, comorbidities, nutrition. Within each of these broad categories the FNP brainstorms all possible causes.

Conclusion

Upon completion of the fishbone diagram, the FNP investigated further into the list of psychiatric medications, and with the consultation of the local hospital physicians, it was concluded the septicemia was due to side effects of the use of psychiatric medications (Depakote, clozapine, fluvoxamine, Seroquel [high dose]). A diagnosis of neuroleptic malignant syndrome was confirmed.

Example Process Map for the APN Leader

Clinical Scenario

A nurse leader managing a medical surgical floor had an increased incidence of patients suffering strokes within 36 hours of transfer for the operating recovery unit. The unit cares for many postop patients from various surgical procedures. After discussing the adverse events with the staff nurses, the nurse leader discovered each of the three patients was diagnosed with pulmonary embolism and started on weight-based heparin protocol infusions. Each patient developed one or more symptoms of persistent headaches, nosebleeds, and "not feeling right." Each of the staff nurses responded by discontinuing the heparin after assessing the patient, only to find the incorrect concentration of heparin was being infused. CT scans were ordered, and each patient had abnormally high partial thromboplastin times, and diagnoses of stroke were confirmed, requiring all three patients to be transferred to intensive care.

The nurse leader knows further analysis of the incidence must be performed and wants to do so through an objective and systematic approach. The nurse leader uses a process map.

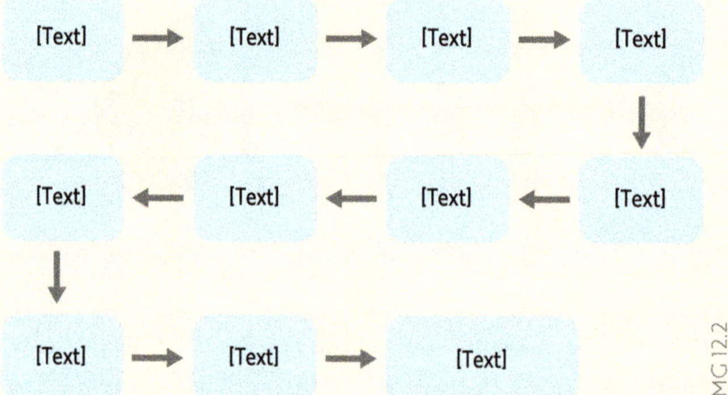

Each box of the process map showed each event, from diagnosis of pulmonary emboli to infusion of heparin and diagnosis of stroke. As a sentinel event, the nurse leader understands the gravity of exploring each event to determine root causes.

Conclusion

As a result of the systematic approach, the nurse leader determined the shipments of heparin from the manufacturer were incorrect, the pharmacy did not identify the error, the medication was correctly labeled but the incorrect concentration was dispensed, the protocol was not double checked, and the incorrect concentration was manually entered into the infusion device.

Example Fishbone Diagram for the APN Educator

Clinical Scenario

Nurse educator faculty in a prelicensure nursing program are concerned due to a continuing decrease in national licensure pass rates. Over the last 3 years and despite efforts to crosswalk the curriculum to the NCLEX blueprint, pass rates fell on average of 3%–5%. The chair of the curriculum committee suggested the use of an RCA tool to begin the process of outcomes evaluation from course to course. They decided on using a fishbone diagram to objectively look at potential root causes in each course and, upon evaluation of each course, as a program.

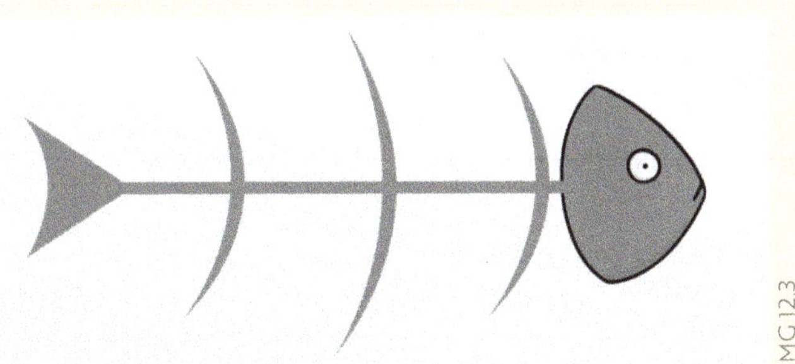

Due to the variation of each course's content and placement in the program, what categories to use for each diagram had to be decided. Each bone was labeled with components of a nursing course, such as materials, clinical experiences, student resources, and teaching strategies.

Conclusion

Upon completion of the fishbone diagram, the nurse educators were able to identify patterns and themes that could be addressed to further support and offer evidence-based teaching strategies that aligned to student learning preferences.

Organize Thinking

The unrestricted and unbiased process from metacognition is just the beginning. As the APN moves to the next phase of the MetaPORT algorithm, organizing thinking is the next step. Most often this phase is done through summarization. To approach this effort, a thinking diary is suggested. In a thinking diary the APN is able to compile and sort the outcomes of the meta-cognition phase from how effective efforts were in calming the mind, reflection, and SWOT analysis, combined with results from problem identification. The review of literature will offer insights into what is known on a professional level, and the RCA method gives personalized insights into the problem/issue. Options for a diary include a written notebook, computer-designed document, or an audio (visual) recording of self. A great deal of good work has already been done by the APN, and therefore deserves to be collected and summarized to assist the APN with filling in memory gaps while highlighting important facts.

A major goal for the thinking diary is to offer summaries of each previous phase of the algorithm. In particular, adding any domino effects can be insightful and lead to innovative solutions. Oftentimes when in the midst of a problem/issue, the effects can be lost or misinterpreted. These domino effects can be highlighted for future considerations. Part of the effort in the thinking diary is to set apart concepts and other issues/topics discovered, which may provide the APN a connection to a nursing theory/model.

Example of a Thinking Diary

An APN clinician is working with a vulnerable population in a rural setting. Resources are scarce, and the APN wants to find solutions to engage the community in topics related to disease prevention and wellness. The APN discovered the following topics in their thinking diary.

Topics/Issues	Concepts Linked to Nursing Theory	Possible Nursing Theory Alignment
Health literacy	Interaction, education, communication	Peplau's interpersonal relations theory

Organizing outcomes can also have personal benefits, much like journaling. The act of documenting thoughts can decrease stress about the situation and improve the outlook for solutions while creating a place for critical thinking. The thinking diary can also be a place to assess the personal efforts of reflection. In this effort, the APN can unlock potential biases that may deter effective (possible) solutions. In addition, the APN can discover new skills/characteristics about themselves and witness their own professional and personal growth.

Relationship to Nursing Theory

A key component to the MetaPORT algorithm is to employ the next phase: relationship to nursing theory. The APN's effort to this point have set the groundwork for identification, analysis, and alignment of a nursing theory or model to assist in creating solutions. The thinking diary can be an effective tool to identify key terms, concepts, topics, and issues, which can then be aligned to major theoretical assumptions. As the text has demonstrated, nursing theory offers more than a foundation of what it is nurses do; it also offers a launching point for finding solutions that are evidence based, safe, and practical and yet still inspire future nursing contributions to health care, leadership, and education.

Nursing theory and models are not as abstract as many of us once thought. Discovering a relationship between the APN clinician, leader, and educator and nursing theory can be a welcome process that offers the APN a sense of not feeling alone or distanced from practicing. Through the grounding nature of theory, APNs can be a guiding light in a health care environment that is complex and ever changing.

Integrative review	+	RCA	+	Summaries (Thinking diary)	+	Highlighted topics	→	Nursing theoretical connections
Apply themes/ patterns of studies examining neuroleptic malignant syndrome		• Lack of full medication reconciliation process • Missing hand-off reports/ documentation • Missed differential diagnosis		Lack of education of neuroleptic syndrome for the FNP/care in the long-term setting		• Interdisciplinary collaborative care • Communication • Education • Holistic assessment		• Lydia E. Hall, *Contribution to Nursing Theory: Care, Cure, Core Theory of Nursing* • Faye Glenn Abdellah, *Contribution to Nursing Theory: Twenty-One Nursing Problems* • Martha E. Rogers, *Contribution to Nursing Theory: Science of Unitary Human Beings*

FIGURE 12.3 Using MetaPORT to align nursing theory/template and example from fishbone diagram for the APN clinician.

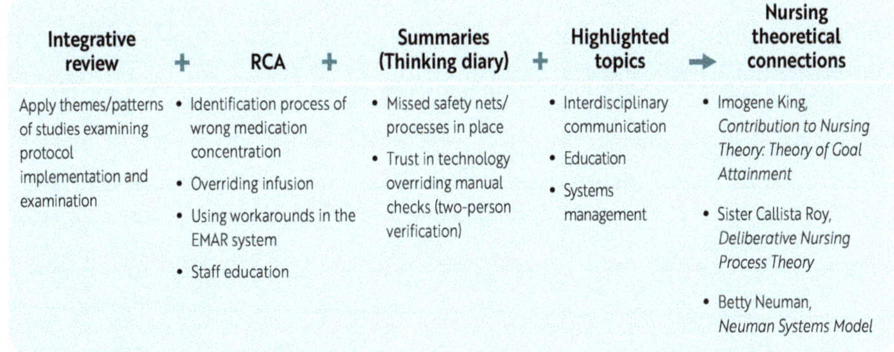

Integrative review	+	RCA	+	Summaries (Thinking diary)	+	Highlighted topics	→	Nursing theoretical connections
Apply themes/patterns of studies examining protocol implementation and examination		• Identification process of wrong medication concentration • Overriding infusion • Using workarounds in the EMAR system • Staff education		• Missed safety nets/ processes in place • Trust in technology overriding manual checks (two-person verification)		• Interdisciplinary communication • Education • Systems management		• Imogene King, *Contribution to Nursing Theory: Theory of Goal Attainment* • Sister Callista Roy, *Deliberative Nursing Process Theory* • Betty Neuman, *Neuman Systems Model*

FIGURE 12.4 Using MetaPORT to align nursing theory/template and example from process map for the APN leader.

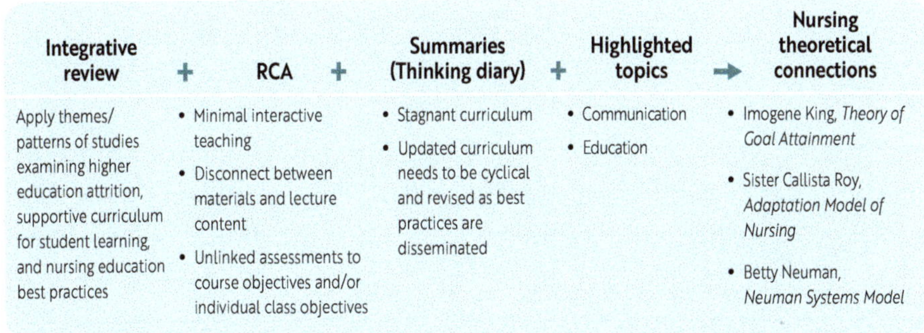

Integrative review	+	RCA	+	Summaries (Thinking diary)	+	Highlighted topics	→	Nursing theoretical connections
Apply themes/ patterns of studies examining higher education attrition, supportive curriculum for student learning, and nursing education best practices		• Minimal interactive teaching • Disconnect between materials and lecture content • Unlinked assessments to course objectives and/or individual class objectives		• Stagnant curriculum • Updated curriculum needs to be cyclical and revised as best practices are disseminated		• Communication • Education		• Imogene King, *Theory of Goal Attainment* • Sister Callista Roy, *Adaptation Model of Nursing* • Betty Neuman, *Neuman Systems Model*

FIGURE 12.5 Using MetaPORT to align nursing theory/template and example from process map for the APN leader.

Talk Out Loud

In the final phase of the MetaPORT algorithm, the APN engages with fellow nursing colleagues and interdisciplinary team members to adopt a CoP. This phase encourages the APN to talk out loud about the process of finding cause/effect and possible solutions while inviting other perspectives relevant to the issue (topic). The act of engaging with others within the same professional environment opens the landscape for learning and sharing information. An area nursing has been historically weak in is in dissemination of knowledge.

Knowledge is a primary source of growth for individuals as well as systems (organizations). Health care is persistently in a state of competition with the need to be highly efficient and sustainable while not compromising quality and safety. Physicians, APNs, nurses, pharmacists, leaders, educators, therapists, and social workers have to leverage their expertise to collaborate with other professionals to solve problems collaboratively, so there is a strong demand for knowledge sharing (Wu et al., 2021). The pressures of each APN role can be overwhelming. With social engagement and collaboration occurring from within a CoP, APN goals, professional satisfaction and continuous learning can thrive.

Figure Credits

IMG 12.1: Source: https://justfreeslide.com/download/free-blank-fishbone-diagram/.
IMG 12.3: Source: https://justfreeslide.com/download/free-blank-fishbone-diagram/.

CHAPTER 13

Aiding Innovative Solutions

Introduction

MetaPORT offers a systematic approach to align knowledge, experience, and evidence to nursing theory; the ultimate goal is to find solutions. Health care is dynamic. The constant flux of new diagnoses, complex care needs, VBC initiatives, and competitive education place the APN in an exceptional position to impact how care is delivered, managed, and taught. It is the intent of this text to inspire APNs to enhance the nursing profession while simultaneously fulfilling professional career satisfaction by practicing to the full extent of their academic preparations. A review of nursing theory's contributions, the APNs unique roles, and a call for innovation is offered.

Nursing Theory Contributions

Nursing theory is the foundation of the profession. Nursing theorists have looked to other disciplines while closely examining the nature of nursing work to create a framework to define the profession. For decades, nursing was unable to describe their actions, but with the development of nursing theories and models, nursing is defined through its practice. As health care and educational environments become more complex, the nursing profession must meet these challenges to maintain its footing while expanding its body of knowledge. The AACN (2021) has revised the "Essentials for Professional Nursing Education" to narrow the gap between nursing research, education, and practice. It is through these recommendations that theory remains essential to grounding future nursing generations to the science of nursing. Looking to the past and noting contributions to nursing practice led by theory is a critical element for the APN to consider as they progress in their academic preparations to be a leader in health care and education.

TABLE 13.1 Examples of Nursing Theory and Its Contributions Over Time

Nursing Theory	Major Theoretical Assumptions	Contributions to Health Care
Nightingale's Environmental Theory **(1860s)**	Environmental principles of fresh air, pure water, efficient drainage, cleanliness, and sunlight all impact human health.	Nightingale's practice of sanitation led to the foundational principle to maintain a clean environment and surroundings at all times when caring for others (patients).
Abdellah's Patient-Centered Approach to Nursing **(1940s)**	Know the patient; organize data; validate the patient's perceptions of their problems; involve the patient and family in care/planning.	Major health care systems employ patient-centered care concepts and practices in their value and mission.
Orem's Self-Care Deficit Theory **(1960s)**	Goal is focused on self-care in that self-efficacy is supported for the patient to participate in care from recovery through maintenance.	Adopt an aim for all levels of care, from primary to tertiary, to gain patient independence.
Kolcaba's Theory of Comfort **(1990s)**	Comfort is an immediate need for patients and an intentional goal for nursing.	Holism, or caring for the patient in a multidimensional way, includes nursing interventions to create comfort and ease pain along the patient's health journey.

Review of the APN's Roles

As laid out in this text, the APN has a wide range of expertise and roles. From clinician to leader and to educator, the APN is uniquely qualified to be a problem solver and spearhead the profession toward the future, with a firm foundation in nursing theory. A final examination of each role, along with a discussion on the possibilities for growth, are important as the APN prepares to take the next steps in their nursing career.

APN Clinician

Nurse practitioners across many specialty practice areas remain steadfast in being recognized for their work and contributions to quality patient care and outcomes. This is evident in the 26 out of 50 states who have adopted full practice authority. Without doubt, NPs will continue to persevere until all 50 states use NPs to the fullest of their education, experience, and expertise.

The demand for NPs continues to grow post-pandemic. To put into context, 355,000 licensed NPs in the United States conduct more than 1 billion patient visits annually, including mobile outreach and telehealth (American Association of Nurse Practitioners, 2023). The NP field is expected to grow nearly 46% by 2031 (U.S. Bureau of Labor Statistics, 2023). With this growth comes great opportunities for APN clinicians, both nurse practitioners and clinical nurse specialists, to engage in meaningful, evidence-based efforts to manage, educate, and solve many health care issues within their specialty areas. The APN clinician offers quality care through a value-based and focused health care system. The result is a win-win for the patient and health care payment systems. An example includes opportunities for the APN clinician to generate public health literacy to promote disease-prevention strategies, such as immunization for respiratory syncytial virus (RSV) while expanding access, particularly for vulnerable populations (application of Pender's health promotion model).

APN Leader

APN leaders are at the center of influencing policy change. Certified nurse leaders obtain specific education and training to use professional competencies to manage an array of dynamic health care settings, from acute inpatient and behavioral units to subacute care and outpatient clinics. A vast number of competencies are required to oversee complex and ongoing challenges. The pandemic left an imprint that has made the role of the APN leader invaluable now and in the future. With the loss of many nurses, leadership has had to become experts in care coordination, conflict management, and technology and data, and has had to become role models, for quality improvement initiatives. The unique contributions of the APN leader are often unseen as they are not only stewards of financial efficiency but also facilitate outcomes management by being amalgamated in care processes to identify patient and family needs. The care and drive to ensure safety in all care settings is a key characteristic of the APN leader. The opportunities for influencing the direction of health care are within the reach for APN leaders.

APN Educator

The APN educator has taken multiple steps to advance their education and practice skill set to offer instruction and pass nursing knowledge to the next generation of nurses and APNs. The role of the nurse educator is complex. Not only does the nurse educator need to be a Master of Educational pedagogies but also impart nursing science and the art of caring in a manner that promotes the development of critical thinkers fully engaged in quality care practices. As health care fluxes, so does nursing education to remain abreast of practice and skill requirements. The days of "telling" nursing students how to be a nurse are dwindling; rather, nursing education is focusing on supporting the student toward independent clinical judgment as a partner in health care delivery. The opportunities for APN educators to influence next generations of nurses is boundless.

A Call for Innovation

By knowing firsthand, the many complexities of health care settings, the APN clinician, leader, and educator are channels for innovation. APNs have experience working with patients and families from birth through death, and their commitment to continue their education and expand their roles are testaments to who they are as nurses: a professional caregiver with authentic dedication to the wellness of others. Through this dedication is a call for nurses and APNs to use their executive functioning skills and expand nursing knowledge to impact the way care is provided, processes are managed, and education is taught. Nursing theory is core to the process of problem solving and innovation as it grounds the APN to its core principles. Through nursing theoretical frameworks, the APN can be guided to find evidence-based solutions while invigorating quality improvement and nursing research. The nursing profession must remain flexible in the post-pandemic era to continue its evolution and expand its knowledge base. *MetaPORT* is a simple, yet systematic and purposeful approach to support APNs in their efforts to make a difference. Now is the time to brush off our memories of nursing theory and reinvigorate theory's contributions to who we are and why we do what we do!

References

Abdellah, F. G., & Levine E. (1994). *Preparing nursing research in the 21st century: Evolution, methodologies, challenges*. Springer.

Agency for Healthcare Research and Quality. (n.d.). *What is patient experience?* https://www.ahrq.gov/cahps/about-cahps/patient-experience/index.html

Aiken, L. H. (2014). Baccalaureate nurses and hospital outcomes: more evidence. *Med Care, 52*(10), 861–863.

Aiken, L. H., Clarke, S. P., Cheung, R., Sloane, D. M., & Silber, J. H. (2003). Educational levels of hospital nurses and surgical patient mortality. *JAMA, 290*(12), 1617–1623. https://doi.org/10.1001/jama.290.12.1617

Aiken, L. H., Sloane, D. M., Brom, H., Todd, B., Barnes, H., Cimiotti, J. P., Cunningham, R., & McHugh, M. D. (2021). Value of nurse practitioner inpatient hospital staffing. *Medical Care, 59*(10), 857–863. https://doi.org/10.1097/mlr.0000000000001628

Allande-Cussó, R., Fernández-García, E., & Porcel-Gálvez, A. M. (2021). Defining and characterising the nurse–patient relationship: A concept analysis. *Nursing Ethics, 29*(2), 462–484. https://doi.org/10.1177/09697330211046651

Almathami, H. K. Y., Win, K. T., & Vlahu-Gjorgievska, E. (2020). Barriers and facilitators that influence telemedicine-based, real-time, online consultation at patients' homes: Systematic literature review. *Journal of Medical Internet Research, 22*(2), e16407. https://doi.org/10.2196/16407

American Association of Colleges of Nursing. (n.d.a.). *AACN essentials*. https://www.aacnnursing.org/Essentials

American Association of Colleges of Nursing. (n.d.b.). *The impact of education on nursing practice*. https://www.aacnnursing.org/news-information/fact-sheets/impact-of-education

American Association of Colleges of Nursing. (n.d.c.). *New graduate employment data*. https://www.aacnnursing.org/News-Information/Research-Data-Center/Employment/2019

American Association of Colleges of Nursing. (2006). *The essentials of doctoral education for advanced nursing practice*. https://www.aacnnursing.org/Portals/42/Publications/DNPEssentials.pdf

American Association of Colleges of Nursing. (2010). *Task force on research-focused doctorate in nursing*. https://www.aacnnursing.org/Portals/42/Publications/DNP-Essentials.pdf

American Association of Colleges of Nursing. (2011). *The essentials of master's education in nursing*. https://www.aacnnursing.org/Portals/42/Publications/MastersEssentials11.pdf

American Association of Colleges of Nursing. (2013). *White paper on the education and role of the clinical nurse leader*. https://www.aacnnursing.org/Portals/42/News/White-Papers/CNL-Competencies-October-2013.pdf

American Association of Critical Care Nurses. (n.d.). *Synergy model*. https://www.aacn.org/nursing-excellence/aacn-standards/synergy-model

American Association of Critical Care Nurses. (2020). *Moral distress in times of crisis.* https://www.aacn.org/policy-and-advocacy/aacn-position-statement-moral-distress-in-times-of-crisis

American Association of Nurse Practitioners. (2024). *More than 290,000 nurse practitioners licensed in the United States.* https://www.aanp.org/about/all-about-nps/np-fact-sheet

American Association of Nurse Practitioners. (2023, January 18). *Five health care trends to watch in 2023.* https://www.aanp.org/news-feed/five-health-care-trends-to-watch-in-2023

American Association of Nurse Practitioners. (n.d.). *NP fact sheet.* https://www.aanp.org/about/all-about-nps/np-fact-sheet

American Association of Nurse Practitioners. (2023, January 18). *Five health care trends to watch in 2023.* https://www.aanp.org/news-feed/five-health-care-trends-to-watch-in-2023

American Holistic Nursing Association. (n.d.). *What we do.* https://www.ahna.org/About-Us/What-is-Holistic-Nursing

American Hospital Association. (n.d.). *Costs of caring.* https://www.aha.org/costsofcaring

American Medical Association. (2022, February 16). *AMA's return on health: Telehealth framework for practices.* https://www.ama-assn.org/practice-management/digital/amas-return-health-telehealth-framework-practices

American Nurses Association. (2016). *Executive summary: American Nurses Association health risk appraisal.* https://www.nursingworld.org/~4aeeeb/globalassets/practiceandpolicy/work-environment/health--safety/ana-healthriskappraisal-summary_2013-2016.pdf

American Nurses Association. (2017). *Executive summary: American Nurses Association health risk appraisal findings.* https://www.nursingworld.org/~4aeeeb/globalassets/practiceandpolicy/work-environment/health--safety/ana-healthriskappraisalsummary_2013-2016.pdf

American Nurses Association. (2017, October 14). *What is Nursing*? https://www.nursingworld.org/practice-policy/workforce/what-is-nursing

American Nurses Association. (2022, March 1). *New survey data: Younger nurses more negatively impacted by COVID-19.* https://www.nursingworld.org/news/news-releases/2022-news-releases/new-survey-data--younger-nurses-more-likely-to-experience-negative-impacts-from-the-covid-19-pandemic/

Association of College & Research Libraries. (2018). *Information literacy competency standards for nursing.* https://www.ala.org/acrl/standards/nursing

Barker, P. (1996). Chaos and the way of Zen: Psychiatric nursing and the "uncertainty principle." *Journal of Psychiatric and Mental Health Nursing, 3*(4), 235–243. https://doi.org/10.1111/j.1365-2850.1996.tb00117.x

Barker, P. (2003). The tidal model: Psychiatric colonization, recovery and the paradigm shift in mental health care. *International Journal of Mental Health Nursing, 12*(2), 96–102. https://doi.org/10.1046/j.1440-0979.2003.00275.x

Bender, M. (2018). Re-conceptualizing the nursing metaparadigm: Articulating the philosophical ontology of the nursing discipline that orients inquiry and practice. *Nursing Inquiry, 25*(3), e12243. https://doi.org/10.1111/nin.12243

Bender, M., & Feldman, M. S. (2015). A practice theory approach to understanding the interdependency of nursing practice and the environment. *Advances in Nursing Science, 38*(2), 96–109. https://doi.org/10.1097/ans.0000000000000068

Benner, P. (2012). *Educating nurses: A call for radical transformation*—How far have we come? *Journal of Nursing Education, 51*(4), 183–184. https://doi.org/10.3928/01484834-20120402-01

Blumenthal, D., & Abrams, M. K. (2013). Putting aside preconceptions—Time for dialogue among primary care clinicians. *The New England Journal of Medicine, 368*(20), 1933–1934. https://doi.org/10.1056/nejme1303343

Bohr, A., & Memarzadeh, K. (2020). The rise of artificial intelligence in healthcare applications. In A. Bohr & K. Memarzadeh (Eds.), *Artifical intelligence in health care* (pp. 25–60). Elsevier. https://doi.org/10.1016/b978-0-12-818438-7.00002-2

Bommier, C. (2019). L'éthique de la conviction confrontée à la technologie. *Ethics, Medicine and Public Health, 9*, 40–44.

Boren, S. A., & Moxley, D. E. (2015). Systematically reviewing the literature: Building the evidence for health care quality. *PubMed, 112*(1), 58–62. https://pubmed.ncbi.nlm.nih.gov/25812277

Boykin, A., Schoenhofer, S. O., Smith, N., St Jean, J., & Aleman, D. (2003). Transforming practice using a caring-based nursing model. *Nursing Administration Quarterly, 27*(3), 223–230. https://doi.org/10.1097/00006216-200307000-00009

Brown M. I. (1964). Research in the development of nursing theory: The importance of a theoretical framework in nursing research. *Nursing Research, 13*, 109–112.

Brunt, B. A., & Bogdan, B. A. (2023). *Nursing professional development leadership.* StatPearls. https://www.ncbi.nlm.nih.gov/books/NBK519064/

Bulman, C. A., Lathlean, J., & Gobbi, M. (2012). The concept of reflection in nursing: Qualitative findings on student and teacher perspectives. *Nurse Education Today, 32*(5), e8–e13. https://doi.org/10.1016/j.nedt.2011.10.007

Buntin, M. B. (2021). Confronting challenges in the US health care system. *JAMA, 325*(14), 1399. https://doi.org/10.1001/jama.2021.1471

Burns, J. M. (2010). *Leadership.* HarperCollins.

Bush, M. (2018). Addressing the root cause. *North Carolina Medical Journal, 79*(1), 26–29. https://doi.org/10.18043/ncm.79.1.26

Byrne, E. K., & Thatchenkery, T. (2019). Cultivating creative workplaces through mindfulness. *Journal of Organizational Change Management, 32*(1), 15–31. https://doi.org/10.1108/jocm-10-2017-0387

Catalyst, N. (2017). What is value-based healthcare? *NEJM Catalyst.* https://catalyst.nejm.org/doi/full/10.1056/CAT.17.0558

Carper, B. (1978). Fundamental patterns of knowing in nursing. *Advances in Nursing Science, 1*(1), 13–23.

Catton, H. (2020). Global challenges in health and health care for nurses and midwives everywhere. *International Nursing Review, 67*(1), 4–6. https://doi.org/10.1111/inr.12578

Centers for Medicare & Medicaid Services. (n.d.). *NHE fact sheet.* https://www.cms.gov/data-research/statistics-trends-and-reports/national-health-expenditure-data/nhe-fact-sheet

Chinn, P., & Jacobs, M. (1978). A model for theory development in nursing. *Advances in Nursing Science, 1*(1), 1–11.

Chinn, P. L., & Kramer, M. K. (2018). *Knowledge development in nursing: Theory and process* (10th ed.). Elsevier.

Christopher. (2020). What is artificial intelligence? How does AI work? *Medium*. https://medium.com/technology-innovations-insights/what-is-artificial-intelligence-how-does-ai-work-585f2d2fdde5

Clark, D. A. (2013). Cognitive restructuring. In S. G. Hoffman, D. J. A. Dozois, W. Rief, & J. Smits (Eds.), *The Wiley handbook of cognitive behavioral therapy* (pp. 1–22). Wiley.

CMS.gov. (2020, March 17). *Medicare telemedicine health care provider fact sheet*. https://www.cms.gov/newsroom/fact-sheets/medicare-telemedicine-health-care-provider-fact-sheet

Colley, S. (2003). Nursing theory: Its importance to practice. *Nursing Standard, 17*(46), 33–37.

Conn, V. S., Isaramalai, S., Rath, S., Jantarakupt, P., Wadhawan, R., & Dash, Y. (2003). Beyond MEDLINE for literature searches. *Journal of Nursing Scholarship, 35*(2), 177–182. https://doi.org/10.1111/j.1547-5069.2003.00177.x

Contreras, J. A., Edwards-Maddox, S., Hall, A. M., & Lee, M. (2020). Effects of reflective practice on baccalaureate nursing students' stress, anxiety and competency: An integrative review. *Worldviews on Evidence-Based Nursing, 17*(3), 239–245. https://doi.org/10.1111/wvn.12438

Cox, C., Amin, K., & Kamal, R. (2021, March 22). *How have health spending and utilization changed during the coronavirus pandemic?* Peterson-KFF Health System Tracker. https://www.healthsystemtracker.org/chart-collection/how-have-healthcare-utilization-and-spending-changed-so-far-during-the-coronavirus-pandemic/

Cross, R. (2020). Understanding the importance of concepts of health. *PubMed, 35*(12), 61–65. 10.7748/ns.2020.e11539

Davis, L., Taylor, H., & Reyes, H. (2014). Lifelong learning in nursing: A Delphi study. *Nurse Education Today, 34*(3), 441–445. https://doi.org/10.1016/j.nedt.2013.04.014

Day L. (2017). The role of theory in nursing education research. In B. J. Patterson & A. M. Krouse (Eds.), *Scientific inquiry in nursing education: Advancing the science* (pp. 13–23). National League for Nursing.

Doyle, C., Lennox, L., & Bell, D. (2013). A systematic review of evidence on the links between patient experience and clinical safety and effectiveness. *BMJ Open, 3*(1), e001570. https://doi.org/10.1136/bmjopen-2012-001570

Dreyfus, S. E. (1982) Formal models vs. human situational understanding: Inherent limitations on the modeling of business expertise. *Office: Technology and People, 1*, 133–155.

Dunlosky, J., & Metcalfe, J. (2008). *Metacognition*. SAGE.

Dunlosky, J., & Thiede, K. W. (1998). What makes people study more? An evaluation of factors that affect self-paced study. *Acta Psychologica, 98*(1), 37–56.

Fawcett J. (1980). A framework for analysis and evaluation of conceptual models of nursing. *Nurse Educator, 5*, 10–14.

Fawcett, J. (2000). *Analysis and evaluation of contemporary nursing knowledge: Nursing models and theories* (3rd ed.). F. A. Davis.

Fine, G., & Burnyeat, M. F. (1992). The Theaetetus of Plato. *The Philosophical Review, 101*(4), 830. https://doi.org/10.2307/2185927

Fitzpatrick, L., Sikka, N., Underwood, K., & HIMSS Global Health Equity Network Collaborators. (2021, November 24). *The digital divide in healthcare: It's not just access*. HIMSS. https://www.himss.org/resources/digital-divide-healthcare-its-not-just-access

Flaskerud, J. H., & Halloran, E. J. (1980). Areas of agreement in nursing theory development. *Advances in Nursing Science, 3*(1), 1–7.

Flavell, J. H. (1979). Metacognition and cognitive monitoring: A new area of cognitive-developmental inquiry. *American Psychologist, 34*(10), 906–911. https://doi.org/10.1037/0003-066x.34.10.906

Fleur, D. S., Bredeweg, B., & Van Den Bos, W. (2021). Metacognition: Ideas and insights from neuro- and educational sciences. *NPJ: Science of Learning, 6*(1). https://doi.org/10.1038/s41539-021-00089-5

Fowler, K. R., & Robbins, L. K. (2022). The impact of COVID-19 on nurse leadership characteristics. *Worldviews on Evidence-Based Nursing, 19*(4), 306–315. https://doi.org/10.1111/wvn.12597

Galanis, P., Vraka, I., Fragkou, D., Bilali, A., & Kaitelidou, D. (2021). Nurses' burnout and associated risk factors during the COVID-19 pandemic: A systematic review and meta-analysis. *Journal of Advanced Nursing, 77*(8), 3286–3302. https://doi.org/10.1111/jan.14839

Godoy, M. (2020, May 30). *What do coronavirus racial disparities look like state by state?* NPR. https://www.npr.org/sections/health-shots/2020/05/30/865413079/what-do-coronavirus-racial-disparities-look-like-state-by-state

Graff-Radford, M. (2022, October 4). Stop practice: A mindfulness technique. *Connect.* Mayo Clinic. https://connect.mayoclinic.org/blog/living-with-mild-cognitive-impairment-mci/newsfeed-post/stop-practice-a-mindfulness-technique/

Grand View Research. (n.d.). *Artificial intelligence in healthcare market size report, 2030.* https://www.grandviewresearch.com/industry-analysis/artificial-intelligence-ai-healthcare-market#:~:text=Artificial%20intelligence%20in%20the%20healthcare%20market%20grew%20at,34.9%25%20to%2048.0%25%20in%20the%20next%205%20years

Grover, A. (2022, August 17). *Health care costs: What's the problem?* Association of American Medical Colleges. https://www.aamc.org/advocacy-policy/aamc-research-and-action-institute/health-care-costs

Haahr, A., Norlyk, A., Martinsen, B., & Dreyer, P. (2019). Nurses experiences of ethical dilemmas: A review. *Nursing Ethics, 27*(1), 258–272. https://doi.org/10.1177/0969733019832941

Hall, L. (1965) Another view of nursing care and quality. In J. George (Ed.), *Nursing theories: The base for professional nursing practice* (pp. 2–12). Appleton & Lange.

Hamric, A. B., Hanson, C. M., Tracy, M. F., & O'Grady, E. T. (2014). *Advanced practice nursing: An integrative approach* (5th ed.). Elsevier.

Han, H. R., Gleason, K. T., Sun, C., Miller, H. N., Kang, S., Chow, S., Anderson, R. C., Nagy, P., & Bauer, T. (2019). Using patient portals to improve patient outcomes: Systematic review. *JMIR Human Factors, 6*(4), e15038. https://doi.org/10.2196/15038

Hassenplug, L. W., & Schlotfeldt, R. M. (1963). Report of the Surgeon General's Consultant Group on nursing. Significance and implications for research in nursing. Nursing research, 12, 68–71.

The Hastings Center. (2023, August 1). *Environment, ethics, and human health.* https://www.thehastingscenter.org/briefingbook/environmental-health/

Healthy People 2030. (n.d.). *Health equity in healthy people 2030.* https://health.gov/healthypeople/priority-areas/health-equity-healthy-people-2030#:~:text=Health%20disparities%20adversely%20affect%20groups,or%20gender%20identity%3B%20geographic%20location%3B

Henderson, V. (1964, August). The nature of nursing. *The American Journal of Nursing, 64*(8), 62–68. https://doi.org/10.2307/3419278

Henderson, V. (1966). The nature of nursing. In George, J. (Ed.), N*ursing theories: the base for professional nursing practice* (pp. 1–84). Appleton & Lange.

Henderson, V. (1978). The concept of nursing. *Journal of Advanced Nursing, 5*, 113–130.

Henderson V. (2006). The concept of nursing. *Journal of Advanced Nursing, 53*(1), 21–31.

Holm, A. L., & Severinsson, E. (2013). Reflections on the ethical dilemmas involved in promoting self-management. *Nursing Ethics, 21*(4), 402–413. https://doi.org/10.1177/0969733013500806

Horsfall, J., Cleary, M., & Hunt, G. E. (2012). Developing a pedagogy for nursing teaching–learning. *Nurse Education Today, 32*(8), 930–933. https://doi.org/10.1016/j.nedt.2011.10.022

Hughes, V. (2018). What are the Barriers to Effective Nurse Leadership? A Review. *Athens Journal of Health, 5*(1), 7–20. https://doi.org/10.30958/ajh.5-1-1

IGI Global. (n.d.). *What is health consumer?* https://www.igi-global.com/dictionary/empirical-study-patient-willingness-use/33258

Institute for Healthcare Improvement. (n.d.). *Triple aim and population health.* https://www.ihi.org/Engage/Initiatives/TripleAim/Pages/default.aspx

Institute of Medicine. (2011). *The future of nursing.* National Academies Press. https://doi.org/10.17226/12956

International Council of Nurses. (2020). *2020 guidelines on advanced practice nursing.*

Interprofessional Education Collaborative. (2016). *Core competencies for interprofessional collaborative practice.* https://ipe.utoronto.ca/sites/default/files/inline-files/IPEC%20Competencies%20Summary%202016.pdf

Jain, A., Leka, S., & Zwetsloot, G. I. (2018). Responsible and ethical business practices and their synergies with health, safety and well-being. In *Aligning perspectives on health, safety and well-being* (pp. 99–138). Springer. https://doi.org/10.1007/978-94-024-1261-1_4

Jha, A. P., Morrison, A. B., Dainer-Best, J., Parker, S. L., Rostrup, N., & Stanley, E. (2015). Minds "at attention": Mindfulness training curbs attentional lapses in military cohorts. *PLOS One, 10*(2), e0116889. https://doi.org/10.1371/journal.pone.0116889

Johns Hopkins Coronavirus Resource Center. (n.d.). *COVID-19 map.* https://coronavirus.jhu.edu/map.html

Johnson, D. E. (1959). The nature of a science of nursing. *Nursing Outlook, 7*(5), 291–294.

Johnson, E., & Carrington, J. M. (2022). Revisiting the nursing metaparadigm: Acknowledging technology as foundational to progressing nursing knowledge. *Nursing Inquiry, 30*(1), e12502. https://doi.org/10.1111/nin.12502

Jun, J. W., Ojemeni, M. T., Kalamani, R., Tong, J., & Crecelius, M. L. (2021). Relationship between nurse burnout, patient and organizational outcomes: Systematic review. *International Journal of Nursing Studies, 119.* https://doi.org/10.1016/j.ijnurstu.2021.103933

Kabat-Zinn, J. (2018). *Meditation is not what you think: Mindfulness and why it is so important.* Hachette.

Kellogg, K. M., Hettinger, Z., Shah, M. N., Wears, R. L., Sellers, C. R., Squires, M., & Fairbanks, R. J. (2016). Our current approach to root cause analysis: is it contributing to our failure to improve patient safety? *BMJ Quality & Safety, 26*(5). https://doi.org/10.1136/bmjqs-2016-005991

Kim, H. S. (2010). *The nature of theoretical thinking in nursing* (3rd ed.). Springer.

King, I. (2007). King's conceptual system, theory of goal attainment, and transaction process in the 21st century. *Nursing Science Quarterly, 20*(2), 109–111.

King, I. M. (1971). Toward a theory for nursing. In George, J. (Ed.). *Nursing theories: The base for professional nursing practice* (pp. 1–132). Appleton & Lange.

Kirca, N., & Özcan, Ş. (2022). The effects of nursing care based on Levine's conservation model on fatigue, depression, perceived social support, and sleep quality in infertile women: A randomized controlled trial. *International Journal of Nursing Knowledge, 34*(4), 284–296. https://doi.org/10.1111/2047-3095.12402

Klein, C. J., Dalstrom, M., Weinzimmer, L. G., Cooling, M., Pierce, L. M., & Lizer, S. (2020). Strategies of advanced practice providers to reduce stress at work. *AAOHN Journal, 68*(9), 432–442. https://doi.org/10.1177/2165079920924060

Knox, M., Willard-Grace, R., Huang, B., & Grumbach, K. (2018). Maslach Burnout Inventory and a self-defined, single-item burnout measure produce different clinician and staff burnout estimates. *Journal of General Internal Medicine, 33*(8), 1344–1351. https://doi.org/10.1007/s11606-018-4507-6

Kooli, C. (2021). COVID-19: Public health issues and ethical dilemmas. *Ethics, Medicine and Public Health, 17.* https://doi.org/10.1016/j.jemep.2021.100635

Koonin, L. M., Hoots, B. E., Tsang, C. A., Leroy, Z., Farris, K., Jolly, T., Antall, P. M., McCabe, B. K., Zelis, C. B. R., Tong, I., & Harris, A. M. (2020). Trends in the use of telehealth during the emergence of the COVID-19 pandemic—United States, January–March 2020. *Morbidity and Mortality Weekly Report, 69*(43), 1595–1599. https://doi.org/10.15585/mmwr.mm6943a3

Krishnan, V. R. (2005). Transformational leadership and outcomes: role of relationship duration. *Leadership & Organization Development Journal, 26*(6), 442–457. https://doi.org/10.1108/01437730510617654

Kruse, C. S., Krowski, N., Rodriguez, B., Tran, L. M., Vela, J., & Brooks, M. L. (2017). Telehealth and patient satisfaction: A systematic review and narrative analysis. *BMJ Open, 7*(8), e016242. https://doi.org/10.1136/bmjopen-2017-016242

Kurtzman, E. T., & Barnow, B. S. (2017). A comparison of nurse practitioners, physician assistants, and primary care physicians' patterns of practice and quality of care in health centers. *Medical Care, 55*(6), 615–622. https://doi.org/10.1097/mlr.0000000000000689

Larson, E., Sharma, J., Bohren, M. A., & Tunçalp, Ö. (2019). When the patient is the expert: Measuring patient experience and satisfaction with care. *Bulletin of the World Health Organization, 97*(8), 563–569. https://doi.org/10.2471/blt.18.225201

Lasater, K. B., Germack, H. D., Small D. S., & McHugh, M. D. (2016). Hospitals known for nursing excellence perform better on value-based purchasing measures. *Policy, Politics, & Nursing Practice, 17*(4), 177–186.

Laurant, M., Van Der Biezen, M., Wijers, N., Watananirun, K., Kontopantelis, E., & Van Vught, A. (2018). Nurses as substitutes for doctors in primary care. *The Cochrane Library, 2019*(2). https://doi.org/10.1002/14651858.cd001271.pub3

Leininger, M. (1999). What is transcultural nursing and culturally competent care? *Journal of Transcultural Nursing, 10*(1). https://doi.org/10.1177/104365969901000105

Leininger, M. (2002). Culture care theory: A major contribution to advance transcultural nursing knowledge and practices. *Journal of Transcultural Nursing 13*, 189–192.

Leininger, M. M., & Mcfarland, M. R. (2002). *Transcultural nursing: Concepts, theories, research, and practice* (3rd ed.). McGraw-Hill.

Letendre, M. (2015). Organizational ethics [Retracted chapter]. In H. ten Have (Ed.), *Encyclopedia of global bioethics* (p. 1). Springer. https://doi.org/10.1007/978-3-319-05544-2_320-1

Levine, M. E. (1967). The four conservation principles of nursing. *Nursing Forum, 6*(1), 45–59. https://doi.org/10.1111/j.1744-6198.1967.tb01297.x

Levine, M. E. (1995). The rhetoric of nursing theory. *Image: The Journal of Nursing Scholarship, 27*(1), 11–14. https://doi.org/10.1111/j.1547-5069.1995.tb00807.x

Linton, M., & Koonmen, J. (2020). Self-care as an ethical obligation for nurses. *Nursing Ethics, 27*(8), 1694–1702. https://doi.org/10.1177/0969733020940371

Lopes, L., Kearney, A., Montero, A., & Brodie, M. (2022, June 16). *Health care debt in the U.S.: The broad consequences of medical and dental bills.* Kaiser Family Foundation. https://www.kff.org/report-section/kff-health-care-debt-survey-main-findings/

Lopes, L., Montero, A., Presiado, M., & Hamel, L. (2022, July 14). *Americans' challenges with health care costs.* Kaiser Family Foundation. https://www.kff.org/health-costs/issue-brief/americans-challenges-with-health-care-costs/

Lovett, M. C. (2008). *Teaching metacognition* [PowerPoint slides]. The University of Rhode Island, Office for the Advancement of Teaching and Learning. http://web.uri.edu/teach/files/Metacognition-ELI.pdf

Lusiyana, A., Yetti, K., & Kuntarti, K. (2019). The strategies of bureaucratic caring implementation by nurse manager: A systematic review. *Enfermería Clínica.* https://doi.org/10.1016/j.enfcli.2019.05.003

Lythreatis, S., El-Kassar, A., & Singh, S. (2021). The digital divide: A review and future research agenda. *Technological Forecasting and Social Change, 175.* https://www.sciencedirect.com/science/article/abs/pii/S0040162521007903

Majerol, M., & Carroll, W. (2018, September 7). *Medicaid and digital health.* Deloitte Insights. https://www2.deloitte.com/us/en/insights/industry/public-sector/mobile-health-care-app-features-for-patients.html

Malinski, V. M. (2022). Unitary human-environment field mutual process: Knowing participation in patterning the environment. *Nursing Science Quarterly, 35*(2), 176–183. https://doi.org/10.1177/08943184211070603

Mambrol, N. (2020, November 9). Cognitive, constructivist learning. *Literary Theory and Criticism.* https://literariness.org/2020/11/09/cognitive-constructivist-learning/

Martinsen, K. (1991). Care and power, words and body in nursing. *Sykepleien [Nursing], 2,* 2–11, 29.

Martinsen, K. (2006). *Care and vulnerability.* Akribe.

Marudhar, M., & Josfeena, M. (2019). Roy's adaptation model of nursing. *International Journal of Scientific Development and Research (IJSDR), 4*(1), 283–285. https://www.ijsdr.org/papers/IJSDR1901049.pdf

Maslow, A. (n.d.). *Self-actualization and beyond.* https://eric.ed.gov/?id=ED012056

MedlinePlus Medical Encyclopedia. (n.d.). *Patient portals.* https://medlineplus.gov/ency/patientinstructions/000880.htm#:~:text=A%20patient%20portal%20is%20a%20website%20for%20your,the%20portal.%20Many%20providers%20now%20offer%20patient%20portals

Meleis, A. I. (2007). *Theoretical nursing: Development and Progress.* Lippincott Williams & Wilkins.

Meleis, A. I. (2011). *Theoretical nursing: Development and Progress.* Lippincott Williams & Wilkins.

Meleis, A. I., Sawyer, L. C., Im, E., Messias, D. K. H., & Schumacher, K. L. (2000). Experiencing transitions: An emerging middle-range theory. *Advances in Nursing Science, 23*(1), 12–28. https://doi.org/10.1097/00012272-200009000-00006

Membrive-Jiménez, M. J., Velando-Soriano, A., Pradas-Hernandez, L., Gómez-Urquiza, J. L., Romero-Béjar, J. L., La Fuente, G. a. C., & De La Fuente-Solana, E. I. (2022). Prevalence, levels and related factors of burnout in nurse managers: A multi-centre cross-sectional study. *Journal of Nursing Management, 30*(4), 954–961. https://doi.org/10.1111/jonm.13575

Mental Health Foundation. (n.d.). What is well-being, how can we measure it and how can we support people to improve it? *Explore Mental Health.* https://www.mentalhealth.org.uk/explore-mental-health/blogs/what-well-being-how-can-we-measure-it-and-how-can-we-support-people-improve-it

Min, D., Lee, J., & Ahn, J. (2023). A qualitative study on the self-care experiences of people with heart failure. *Western Journal of Nursing Research, 45*(7), 646–652. https://doi.org/10.1177/01939459231169102

Mishel, M. H. (1983). Adjusting the fit: Development of uncertainty scales for specific clinical populations. *Western Journal of Nursing Research 5*(4), 355–370.

Mishel, M. H. (1988). Uncertainty in illness. *Journal of Nursing Scholarship, 20*(4), 225–232. https://doi.org/10.1111/j.1547-5069.1988.tb00082.x

Molina-Mula, J., & Gallo-Estrada, J. (2020). Impact of nurse-patient relationship on quality of care and patient autonomy in decision-making. *International Journal of Environmental Research and Public Health, 17*(3), 835. https://doi.org/10.3390/ijerph17030835

Monaro, S., Pinkova, J., Ko, N., Stromsmoe, N., & Gullick, J. (2021). Chronic wound care delivery in wound clinics, community nursing and residential aged care settings: A qualitative analysis using Levine's conservation model. *Journal of Clinical Nursing, 30*(9–10), 1295–1311. https://doi.org/10.1111/jocn.15674

Nana-Sinkam, P., Kraschnewski, J. L., Sacco, R. L., Chavez, J. V., Fouad, M. N., Gal, T. S., AuYoung, M., Namoos, A., Winn, R. A., Sheppard, V. B., Corbie-Smith, G., & Behar-Zusman, V. (2021). Health disparities and equity in the era of COVID-19. *Journal of Clinical and Translational Science, 5*(1). https://doi.org/10.1017/cts.2021.23

Nancarrow, S., Booth, A., Ariss, S., Smith, T. P., Enderby, P., & Roots, A. (2013). Ten principles of good interdisciplinary teamwork. *Human Resources for Health, 11*(1). https://doi.org/10.1186/1478-4491-11-19

The National Academies of Sciences, Engineering, and Medicine. (2017). *Communities in action: Pathways to health equity.* National Academies Press.

The National Academies of Sciences, Engineering, and Medicine (2019). *Integrating social care into the delivery of health care: Moving upstream to improve the nation's health.* National Academies Press.

National Academies of Sciences, Engineering, and Medicine, National Academy of Medicine, Flaubert, J. L., Menestrel, L. S., Williams, D. R., & Wakefield, M. K. (2021, September 11). *The future of nursing 2020–2030: Charting a path to achieve health equity.* National Academies Press.

National Advisory Council on Nurse Education and Practice. (2021). *Preparing nurse faculty and addressing the shortage of nurse faculty and clinical preceptors.* Health Resources and Services Administration. https://www.hrsa.gov/sites/default/files/hrsa/advisory-committees/nursing/reports/nacnep-17report-2021.pdf

National Advisory Council on Nurses. (2019). *Promoting nursing leadership in the transition to value-based care.* https://www.hrsa.gov/sites/default/files/hrsa/advisory-committees/nursing/reports/2019-fifteenthreport.pdf

National League for Nursing. (2022, May 16). *Default.* https://www.nln.org/detail-pages/news/2022/05/16/nurse-educators-play-vital-roles-in-health-care

National Organization of Nurse Practitioner Faculties. (2022, March). *National Organization of Nurse Practitioner Faculties' nurse practitioner role core competencies.* https://www.nonpf.org/page/NP_Role_Core_Competencies

Newman, M. A. (1994). *Health as expanding consciousness* (2nd ed.). Jones & Bartlett Learning.

Nightingale, F. (1980). *Notes on nursing: what it is, and what it is not.* https://ci.nii.ac.jp/ncid/BB28458389

Nundy, S. (2021). *Care after Covid: What the pandemic revealed is broken in healthcare and how to reinvent it.* McGraw-Hill.

Oxford English Dictionary Online. (1989). *Authenticity.* https://www.oed.com/?tl=true

Papanicolas, I., Woskie, L., & Jha, A. K. (2018). Health care spending in the United States and other high-income countries. *JAMA, 319*(10), 1024. https://doi.org/10.1001/jama.2018.1150

Papastavrou, E., Acaroğlu, R., Şendir, M., Berg, A., Efstathiou, G., Idvall, E., Kalafati, M., Katajisto, J., Leino-Kilpi, H., Lemonidou, C., Da Luz, M. D. A., & Suhonen, R. (2015). The relationship between individualized care and the practice environment: An international study. *International Journal of Nursing Studies, 52*(1), 121–133. https://doi.org/10.1016/j.ijnurstu.2014.05.008

Parker J. M., & Hill M. N. (2017). A review of advanced practice nursing in the United States, Canada, Australia, and Hong Kong Special Administrative Region (SAR), China. *International Journal of Nursing Sciences, 4*(2), 196–204. https://doi.org/10.1016/j.ijnss.2017.01.002

Patel, K. M., & Metersky, K. (2021). Reflective practice in nursing: A concept analysis. *International Journal of Nursing Knowledge, 33*(3), 180–187. https://doi.org/10.1111/2047-3095.12350

Patient Engagement HIT. (2021, June 21). *How did gaps in hospital quality affect COVID-19 health disparities?* https://patientengagementhit.com/news/how-did-gaps-in-hospital-quality-affect-covid-19-health-disparities

Patterson, B. J. (2021, November). A dynamic relationship between theory and research in nursing education. *Nursing Education Perspectives, 42*(6), 337–338. https://doi.org/10.1097/01.nep.0000000000000903

Peden, A. R. (2018). Letters from Peplau. *Journal of the American Psychiatric Nurses Association, 24*(5), 444–451. https://doi.org/10.1177/1078390318763943

Penque, S. (2019). Mindfulness to promote nurses' well-being. *Nursing Management, 50*(5), 38–44. https://doi.org/10.1097/01.numa.0000557621.42684.c4

Peplau, H. E. (1991). *Interpersonal relations in nursing.* Springer.

Peplau, H. E. (1992). Interpersonal relations: A theoretical framework for application in nursing practice. *Nursing Science Quarterly, 5*(1), 13–18. https://doi.org/10.1177/089431849200500106

Peplau, H. E. (1997). Peplau's theory of interpersonal relations. *Nursing Science Quarterly, 10*(4), 162–167. https://doi.org/10.1177/089431849701000407

Perloff, J., DesRoches, C. M., & Buerhaus, P. I. (2016). Comparing the cost of care provided to Medicare beneficiaries assigned to primary care nurse practitioners and physicians. *Health Services Research, 51*(4), 1407–1423. https://doi.org/10.1111/1475-6773.12425

PestleAnalysis Contributor. (2021, May 30). *What is a simplified SWOT analysis definition in 4 steps.* https://pestleanalysis.com/swot-analysis-definition/

Peterson, S. J. (2013). Interpersonal relations. In S. J. Peterson & T. S. Bredow (Eds.), *Middle range theories: Application to nursing research* (3rd ed., pp. 138–159). Wolters Kluwer/Lippincott, Williams & Wilkins.

Phelan, P. S. (2020). Organizational ethics for US health care today. *AMA Journal of Ethics, 22*(3), E183–E186. https://doi.org/10.1001/amajethics.2020.183

Pharris, M. D. (2011). Margaret A. Newman's theory of health as expanding consciousness. *Nursing Science Quarterly, 24*(3), 193–194. https://doi.org/10.1177/0894318411409437

Philips. (n.d.). *Healthcare hits reset.* https://www.philips.com/a-w/about/news/future-health-index/reports/2022/healthcare-hits-reset

Pruitt, Z., Emechebe, N., Quast, T., Taylor, P. L., & Bryant, K. M. (2018). Expenditure Reductions Associated with a Social Service Referral Program. *Population Health Management, 21*(6), 469–476. https://doi.org/10.1089/pop.2017.0199

Proust, J. (2013). *The philosophy of metacognition: Mental agency and self-awareness.* Oxford University Press.

PYMNTS. (2022, July 26). *Inaccurate cost estimates could push 60% of patients to switch providers.* https://pymnts.com/healthcare-financing/2022/inaccurate-cost-estimates-could-push-60-of-patients-to-switch-providers/

Raghubir, A. E. (2018). Emotional intelligence in professional nursing practice: A concept review using Rodgers's evolutionary analysis approach. *International Journal of Nursing Sciences, 5*(2), 126–130. https://doi.org/10.1016/j.ijnss.2018.03.004

Ransing, R., Ramalho, R., De Filippis, R., Ojeahere, M. I., Karaliūnienė, R., Orsolini, L., Da Costa, M. P., Ullah, I., Grandinetti, P., Bytyçi, D. G., Grigo, O., Mhamunkar, A., Hayek, S. E., Essam, L., Larnaout, A., Shalbafan, M., Nofal, M., Soler-Vidal, J., Pereira-Sánchez, V., & Adiukwu, F. (2020). Infectious disease outbreak related stigma and discrimination during the COVID-19 pandemic: Drivers, facilitators, manifestations, and outcomes across the world. *Brain Behavior and Immunity, 89*, 555–558. https://doi.org/10.1016/j.bbi.2020.07.033

Rasheed, S. P., Sundus, A., Younas, A., Fakhar, J., & Inayat, S. (2020). Development and testing of a measure of self-awareness among nurses. *Western Journal of Nursing Research, 43*(1), 36–44. https://doi.org/10.1177/0193945920923079

Rasheed S. P., Younas A., Sundus A. (2019). Self-awareness in nursing: A scoping review. *Journal of Clinical Nursing, 28*(5–6), 762–774.

Ray, M. A. (1989). The theory of bureaucratic caring for nursing practice in the organizational culture. *Nursing Administration Quarterly, 13*(2), 31–42. https://doi.org/10.1097/00006216-198901320-00007

Richards, A. (2020). Exploring the benefits and limitations of transactional leadership in healthcare. *Nursing Standard, 35*(12), 46–50. https://doi.org/10.7748/ns.2020.e11593

Riegel, F., Crossetti, M. D. G. O., Martini, J. G., & Nes, A. A. G. (2021). Florence Nightingale's theory and her contributions to holistic critical thinking in nursing. *Revista Brasileira de Enfermagem, 74*(2). https://doi.org/10.1590/0034-7167-2020-0139

Rogers, M. (1970b). Introduction to the theoretical basis of nursing. *Nursing Research, 19*(6), 541. https://doi.org/10.1097/00006199-197011000-00012

Rogers, E. M., Simon, H. D., & Schuster. (2003). *Diffusion of Innovations, 5th Edition.* https://www.amazon.com/Diffusion-Innovations-5th-Everett-Rogers/dp/0743258231

Roy, C. (1997). Future of the Roy model: Challenge to redefine adaptation. *Nursing Science Quarterly, 10*(1), 42–48. https://doi.org/10.1177/089431849701000113

Roy, C., Whetsell, M. V., & Frederickson, K. (2009). The Roy adaptation model and research. *Nursing Science Quarterly, 22*(3), 209–211. https://doi.org/10.1177/0894318409338692

Roy, C. (2011). Research based on the Roy adaptation model. *Nursing Science Quarterly, 24*(4), 312–320. https://doi.org/10.1177/0894318411419218

Roy, C. (2011). Extending the Roy adaptation model to meet changing global needs. *Nursing Science Quarterly, 24*, 345–351.

Roy, C., Whetsell, M. V., & Frederickson, K. (2009). The Roy adaptation model and research. *Nursing Science Quarterly*, *22*(3), 209–211. https://doi.org/10.1177/0894318409338692

Saad, B. L. (2023, June 5). *Military brass, judges among professions at new image lows*. Gallup. https://news.gallup.com/poll/388649/military-brass-judges-among-professions-new-image-lows.aspx

Sagar, P. L., & Sagar, D. Y. (2018). Current state of transcultural nursing theories, models, and approaches. *Annual Review of Nursing Research*, *37*(1), 25–41. https://doi.org/10.1891/0739-6686.37.1.25

Schwerdtle, P. N., Connell, C. J., Lee, S., Plummer, V., Russo, P. L., Endacott, R., & Kuhn, L. (2020). Nurse expertise: A critical resource in the COVID-19 pandemic response. *Annals of Global Health*, *86*(1). https://doi.org/10.5334/aogh.2898

Salvage, J., & White, J. (2019). Nursing leadership and health policy: Everybody's business. *International Nursing Review*, *66*(2), 147–150. https://doi.org/10.1111/inr.12523

Scaled Agile Framework. (2020, June 30). *Value streams*. https://www.scaledagileframework.com/value-streams/

Schumacher, K. L., & Meleis, A. I. (1994). Transitions: A central concept in nursing. *Image: The Journal of Nursing Scholarship*, *26*(2), 119–127. https://doi.org/10.1111/j.1547-5069.1994.tb00929.x

Shaver, J. (2022). The state of telehealth before and after the COVID-19 pandemic. *Primary Care*, *49*(4), 517–530. https://doi.org/10.1016/j.pop.2022.04.002

Shea, N. (2019). Concept-metacognition. *Mind & Language*, *35*(5), 565–582. https://doi.org/10.1111/mila.12235

Siegesmund, A. (2017). Using self-assessment to develop metacognition and self-regulated learners. *FEMS Microbiology Letters*, *364*(11). https://doi.org/10.1093/femsle/fnx096

Silver, S., Li, J., Marsh, S., & Carbone, E. (2022, August 29). Pre-pandemic mental health and well-being of healthcare workers. *NIOSH Science*. https://blogs.cdc.gov/niosh-science-blog/2022/08/29/hcw-mental-health-prepandemic/

Slattery, M. J., Logan, B. L., Mudge, B., Secore, K., von Reyn, L. J., & Maue, R. A. (2016). An undergraduate research fellowship program to prepare nursing students for future workforce roles. *Journal of Professional Nursing*, *32*(6), 412–420. https://doi.org/10.1016/j.profnurs.2016.03.008

Steptoe, A., & Marmot, M. (2002). The role of psychobiological pathways in socio-economic inequalities in cardiovascular disease risk. *European Heart Journal*, *23*(1), 13–25. https://doi.org/10.1053/euhj.2001.2611

Stucke, N. (2021, August 16). *Metacognition and executive function: a dynamic relationship of cognitive functioning*. Reflection Sciences. https://reflectionsciences.com/blog-metacognition-executive-function/

Stucky, C. H., Brown, W. J., & Stucky, M. G. (2020). COVID 19: An unprecedented opportunity for nurse practitioners to reform healthcare and advocate for permanent full practice authority. *Nursing Forum*, *56*(1), 222–227. https://doi.org/10.1111/nuf.12515

Sturmberg, J. P., & Bircher, J. (2019). Better and fulfilling healthcare at lower costs: The need to manage health systems as complex adaptive systems. *F1000Research*, *8*, 789. https://doi.org/10.12688/f1000research.19414.1

Sullivan, D. K., Sullivan, V., Weatherspoon, D., & Frazer, C. (2021). Comparison of nurse burnout, before and during the COVID-19 pandemic. *Nursing Clinics of North America*, *57*(1), 79–99. https://doi.org/10.1016/j.cnur.2021.11.006

Swanson, E. (2022, January 31). *National hospital flash report: January 2022.* Kaufman Hall. https://www.kaufmanhall.com/insights/research-report/national-hospital-flash-report-january-2022

Tableau. (n.d.). *Root cause analysis explained: Definition, examples, and methods.* https://www.tableau.com/learn/articles/root-cause-analysis

Telehealth.HHS.gov. (n.d.). *Why use telehealth?* https://telehealth.hhs.gov/patients/understanding-telehealth/

Thompson, W., & McNamara, M. (2021). Constructing the advanced nurse practitioner identity in the healthcare system: A discourse analysis. *Journal of Advanced Nursing, 78*(3), 834–846. https://doi.org/10.1111/jan.15068

Travelbee, J. (1971). *Interpersonal aspects of nursing* (2nd ed.). F. A. Davis Company.

Trilla, F., DeCastro, T., Harrison, N., Mowry, D., Croke, A., Bicket, M., & Buechner, J. (2018). Nurse practitioner home-based primary care program improves patient outcomes. *The Journal for Nurse Practitioners, 14*(9), e185–e188. https://doi.org/10.1016/j.nurpra.2018.08.003

Ulrich, B., Barden, C., Cassidy, L., & Varn-Davis, N. (2019). Frontline nurse manager and chief nurse executive skills: Perceptions of direct care nurses. *Nurse Leader, 17*(2), 109–112. https://doi.org/10.1016/j.mnl.2018.12.014

United Nations. (n.d.). *The 17 goals.* https://sdgs.un.org/goals

U.S. Bureau of Economic Analysis. (n.d.). *Gross domestic product.* https://www.bea.gov/resources/learning-center/what-to-know-gdp

U.S. Bureau of Labor Statistics. (2022, September 8). Registered nurses. *Occupational outlook handbook.* https://www.bls.gov/ooh/healthcare/registered-nurses.htm

U.S. Bureau of Labor Statistics. (2023, September 6). *Fastest growing occupations.* https://www.bls.gov/emp/tables/fastest-growing-occupations.htm

U.S. Department of Health and Human Services, & Cochran, N. (n.d.). FY 2022 Annual Performance Plan and Report. In *FY 2022 Annual Performance Plan and Report* (pp. 2–4). https://www.hhs.gov/sites/default/files/fy2022-performance-plan.pdf

U.S. Government Accountability Office. (2021, September 18). Racial and ethnic health disparities—Before and during the pandemic. *Following the Federal Dollar.* https://www.gao.gov/blog/racial-and-ethnic-health-disparities-and-during-pandemic

Vadivel, R., Shoib, S., Halabi, S. E., Hayek, S. E., Essam, L., Bytyçi, D. G., Karaliūnienė, R., Teixeira, A. L. S., Nagendrappa, S., Ramalho, R., Ransing, R., Pereira-Sánchez, V., Jatchavala, C., Adiukwu, F., & Kundadak, G. K. (2021). Mental health in the post-COVID-19 era: Challenges and the way forward. *General Psychiatry, 34*(1), e100424. https://doi.org/10.1136/gpsych-2020-100424

Van Calster, B., Wynants, L., Timmerman, D., Steyerberg, E. W., & Collins, G. S. (2019). Predictive analytics in health care: how can we know it works? *Journal of the American Medical Informatics Association, 26*(12), 1651–1654. https://doi.org/10.1093/jamia/ocz130

Van Der Riet, P., Levett-Jones, T., & Aquino-Russell, C. (2018). The effectiveness of mindfulness meditation for nurses and nursing students: An integrated literature review. *Nurse Education Today, 65*, 201–211. https://doi.org/10.1016/j.nedt.2018.03.018

Varkey, B. (2020a). Principles of clinical ethics and their application to practice. *Medical Principles and Practice, 30*(1), 17–28. https://doi.org/10.1159/000509119

Vijayaraghavan, M., Tochterman, A. Z., Hsu, E., Johnson, K. C., Marcus, S. M., & Caton, C. L. M. (2011). Health, Access to Health Care, and Health Care use Among Homeless

Women with a History of Intimate Partner Violence. *Journal of Community Health, 37*(5), 1032–1039. https://doi.org/10.1007/s10900-011-9527-7

Waisel, D. B. (2013). Vulnerable populations in healthcare. *Current Opinion in Anesthesiology, 26*(2), 186–192. https://doi.org/10.1097/aco.0b013e32835e8c17

Wang, J., Lim, M. K., Wang, C., & Tseng, M. (2021). The evolution of the Internet of Things (IoT) over the past 20 years. *Computers & Industrial Engineering, 155*. https://doi.org/10.1016/j.cie.2021.107174

Watson, J. (1985). Nursing: Human science and human care. A theory of nursing. *National League for Nursing Publications, 15–2236*, 1–104. https://pubmed.ncbi.nlm.nih.gov/3375032

Watson, J. (2008). *Nursing: The philosophy and science of caring* (Revised ed.). University Press of Colorado.

Watson Caring Science Institute. (2023, September 14). *Watson's caring science & theory*. https://www.watsoncaringscience.org/jean-bio/caring-science-theory/

Weiner, J. P., Sh, B., Hatef, E., Lans, D., Liu, A. M., & Lemke, K. W. (2021). In-person and telehealth ambulatory contacts and costs in a large US insured cohort before and during the COVID-19 pandemic. *JAMA Network Open, 4*(3), e212618. https://doi.org/10.1001/jamanetworkopen.2021.2618

Wiedenbach, E. (1970). Nurses' wisdom in nursing theory. *The American Journal of Nursing, 70*(5), 1057–1062. https://doi.org/10.2307/3421362

Wikipedia contributors. (2023, March 18). *2023*. Wikipedia. https://en.wikipedia.org/wiki/2023

W.K. Kellogg Foundation. (2023, September 19). *Home page*. https://www.wkkf.org/

World Health Organization. (n.d.a). *Constitution*. https://www.who.int/about/governance/constitution#:~:text=Health%20is%20a%20state%20of,absence%20of%20disease%20or%20infirmity

World Health Organization. (n.d.b). *Homepage*. https://www.who.int/

World Health Organization. (2019, May 28). *Burn-out an "occupational phenomenon": International classification of diseases*. https://www.who.int/news/item/28-05-2019-burn-out-an-occupational-phenomenon-international-classification-of-diseases

Wu, S., Wang, W., & Hsiao, M. (2021). Knowledge sharing among healthcare practitioners: Identifying the psychological and motivational facilitating factors. *Frontiers in Psychology, 12*. https://doi.org/10.3389/fpsyg.2021.736277

Yu, K., Beam, A. L., & Kohane, I. S. (2018). Artificial intelligence in healthcare. *Nature Biomedical Engineering, 2*(10), 719–731. https://doi.org/10.1038/s41551-018-0305-z

Index

K

L

M

N

T

U

V

W

www.ingramcontent.com/pod-product-compliance
Ingram Content Group UK Ltd.
Pitfield, Milton Keynes, MK11 3LW, UK
UKHW050140280726
14058UKWH00006B/758